Assessment and Culture

Assessment and Culture

Psychological Tests
with Minority Populations

Sharon-ann Gopaul-McNicol
Eleanor Armour-Thomas

Academic Press

San Diego   London   Boston   New York   Sydney   Tokyo   Toronto

Academic Press
A division of Harcourt, Inc.
525 B Street, Suite 1900, San Diego, California 92101-4495, USA
http://www.academicpress.com

Academic Press
Harcourt Place, 32 Jamestown Road, London NW1 7BY, UK
http://www.academicpress.com

Library of Congress Catalog Card Number: 2001094481

International Standard Book Number: 0-12-290451-6

PRINTED IN THE UNITED STATES OF AMERICA
01 02 03 04 05 06 SB 9 8 7 6 5 4 3 2 1

To our Families—Ulric, Monique, Monica, Bernard,
Renaté and Bianca with Gratitude and Love
And in Loving memory of our Parents
St. Elmo Gopaul and Cleaver and Celita Armour

CONTENTS

PART **III**

Implications for Cross-Cultural
Training, Research, and Policy

PREFACE

This book is the culmination of thirteen years of cross-cultural practice (assessment and treatment), research, consultation and supervision with families of various ethnic and cultural backgrounds. As we developed programs and served as a consultants to various educational and clinical institutions throughout the United States, the United Kingdom, Canada, and the Caribbean, we came to realize that a different approach to assessment is needed if culturally diverse families are to smoothly acculturate in this society.

Our work led us to conclude that a more comprehensive approach to assessment is needed, to best understand the strengths of these diverse populations. The bio-cultural approach to all areas of assessment that we propose here was developed after assessing over 2,500 individuals in the school, clinical, home and community settings, and serving as consultants to practitioners, researchers and teachers in a variety of arenas.

This book introduces a model for assessment—a bio-cultural approach. The principal objective of this model is to help mental health professionals more accurately assess individuals from various ethnic, cultural and linguistic backgrounds. The techniques and strategies proposed by these models are indicative of an eclectic perspective. From a culture-fair perspective, this model allows the examiner the opportunity to tap all of the strengths of the individual being assessed. Besides, humanistically speaking, this approach allows the therapist to view the world through the lenses of the examinee. Finally, from an ethnocultural/ethnopsychological perspective, this model has endorsed the assumption that each cultural set of circumstances results in a unique response and coping style, crucial to one's development.

The theoretical bases for such a comprehensive approach to assessment originated from cross-cultural psychology, cross-cultural mental health with ethnic minorities in the United States and people who come from oppressed systems around the world. As such, this model has several categories where assessment is carried out: standardized, non-standardized potential and in the examinee's ecology. In other words, this model seeks to empower the client through observing their strengths by the manner in which they relate and interact with various systems in the examinee's real world.

Sharon-Ann Gopaul-McNicol
Eleanor Armour-Thomas

ACKNOWLEDGMENTS

To our immediate family, Ulric, Monique Mandisa, Monica Gopaul, Bernard, Renaté, Bianca, we extend our most profound gratitude. Your love, patience and unflagging support throughout this challenging time will be remembered in our hearts forever.

To our parents who instilled in us a sense of confidence and pride about "being the best you can be," we extend much gratitude, respect and tenderness.

To our siblings, Gail, Wendy, Kurt, Nigel, Gail Marie, Felicia, Brenda, Judy, Marcia, Cleavy, Edward, Margaret, our nieces and nephews Michael, Kja, Michelle, Alexis, Skyler, Kris, Ricardo, Brian, Jerry, Paula, Gena, Catrice, Wesley, Reid, our cousins Doreen, Autricia and Maria, we thank you for your on going support and patience.

To our professional colleagues and special friends who have helped to nurture a respect for cross-cultural inquiry, we thank you immensely. In particular, we would like to extend our appreciation to the following individuals— Earl George, Coleen Clay, Brenda Allen, Dawn Arno, Ann Francis-Okongwu, Miriam Azaunce, Norris Haynes, James Williams, Janet Brice-Baker, Randolf Tobias, William Proefriedt, Aldrena Mabry, Nicola Beckles, Lauraine Casella, Arthur Dozier, George Irish, Delroy Louden, Michael Barnes, Alice F. Artzt, Jesse M. Vazquez, Kabba Colley, Yu Ren Dong, Emery Francois, Erika Wick, James Curley, Trevor Davis, Eric Eisen, John Nwogu, Joya Gomez, Charmaine Edwards, Headley Wilson, Susan Lokai, Seretse McHardy, Koreen Seabrun, Sandra Hosein, Jennifer D'Ade, Joanne Julien, Linda Brady, Sharon Albert, Colga Hylton, Cassandra Kemp, Ieshia Haynie, and Ann Carter-Obayuwana.

To our research assistants—Grace Reid, Orlean Brown, Jamila Mitchell, Jacquelyn Gordon, Angela Lee, Kaia Brown, Renaté and Bianca Thomas, and other students in training who provided much support, we extend our gratitude.

To the leading thinkers in the field who most influenced our work—
Edmund W. Gordon, A. Wade Boykin, Jim Cummins, Stephen Ceci, Richard
Dana, Richard Figueroa, Howard Gardner, Janet Helms, Asa Hilliard, Jean
Lave, Ulric Neisser, Esteban Olmedo, Robert Sternberg, Lev Vygotsky, and
Robert Williams, we extend our deepest respect and gratitude.

To the communities and students of the University of the West Indies,
Howard University, Queens College, St. John's University, and the American
Psychological Association, we thank you for your support in the nurturing of
our thinking.

We also express our deepest appreciation to George Zimmar, former Senior
Editor of Academic Press for nurturing this project and for his wise advice.
Our gratitude also extends to Traci John, Production Manager at Academic
Press for her timely reminders on deadlines and her patience in accommodating our last minute changes. We are indebted to both her and the typesetters
at Hermitage Publishing Services for their high quality and efficient work in
attending to the revisions and in putting the manuscript into its finished form.

We would like to thank the publishers who granted us permission to use
segments of our own work from our published journals, book chapters and
books.

To our deceased loved ones, St. Elmo Gopaul, Josephine Fritzgerald,
Cleaver and Celita Armour, and Christopher Edwards, may God bless you all.

PART I

Socio-Political and Ethical Issues in Cross-Cultural Assessment

CHAPTER 1

Introduction

The percentage of individuals who come from culturally and linguistically diverse backgrounds is growing larger in the United States (U.S. Department of Commerce News, 1989). This situation has resulted in an increase in immigration issues and a concerted effort to address the multiplicity and complexity of concerns associated with this process. Historically, the United States had addressed this influx of multiple cultures by expecting everyone to assimilate into the society (the melting pot syndrome), resulting in an expected denouncing of any linguistic and cultural ties. Another way that the preponderance of immigration was dealt with was to marginalize those who attempted, for one reason or another, to maintain their cultural and linguistic affinity.

In conflict with the expected assimilation standard, new immigrant groups from diverse cultural backgrounds are expecting more understanding of their unique cultural and social mores from members of the American society. At the core of the debate is the question: What are the true natures of intelligence, academic achievement, and emotional disturbance, and how can one best measure them? Culturally diverse clients are claiming that their potentials are not being tapped by these standardized measures of assessment. Thus, there is

much misdiagnosis by professionals unfamiliar with their cultural backgrounds and social customs. Therefore, these clients are asking for more relevant programmatic, educational and clinical interventions to meet their educational and social needs. The end result is that the mental health and educational systems are desperately trying to hone their skills to address the needs
of these cultural groups.

In an attempt to prepare mental health workers and educators to address
the educational, social, and emotional needs of the culturally diverse client, we
independently call for a more flexible approach to assessment than the traditional one usually utilized by clinicians and evaluators. In other words, we are
calling for a more multidimensional, dynamic approach, which allows for
more individualistic and ecological information to be included in the diagnostic equation.

This book is divided into three parts. Part I examines the challenges of non-
discriminatory assessment in a culturally diverse society (chapters 1 and 2).
Chapter 3 looks at the ethical and legal issues in cross-cultural assessment.
Chapter 4 proposes a new perspective on assessment—a bio-cultural model
developed by the present authors.

Part II explores practical issues in cross-cultural assessment with chapter 5
focusing on assessing the intellectual functioning of culturally diverse children. Chapter 6 examines linguistic issues in assessing culturally diverse individuals. Chapter 7 looks at how to best assess the academic performance of
culturally diverse children and chapter 8 explores issues in assessing the visual-motor and neurological functioning of culturally diverse children. Assessing
the personality of culturally diverse children is discussed in chapter 9, while
cultural issues in vocational/guidance assessment are examined in chapter 10.
A biocultural approach to report writing is explored in chapter 11.

Part III offers training suggestions for school personnel, teachers and parents for enhancing the intellectual potential of culturally diverse children
(chapter 12). Finally, implications for future research and clinical work, as well
as a vision for policymakers as to how to ensure culturally sensitive assessment
and tutelage, are suggested in chapters 13 and 14.

CHAPTER 2

The Challenge of Non-discriminatory Assessment in a Culturally Diverse Society

INTRODUCTION

The disproportionate number of children from culturally diverse backgrounds in low track classes (Gamoran and Nystrand, 1990; Oakes, 1990), in special education programs (Armour-Thomas, 1992; Gopaul-McNicol, 1992a; Cummins, 1984) and in the psychiatric care system has led many educators and psychologists to question the decision-making that has led to these placements. Usually, decision-making regarding placement of children in these programs is based on results from standardized assessment measures (e.g., tests of intelligence, personality, academic achievement and language proficiency). Proponents of standardized assessments defend them on the grounds that they meet the psychometric criteria of reliability and validity and the purposes for which they were intended: selection, sorting and prediction. However, over the last thirty years, a recurring criticism among many psychologists and educators is that standardized tests are invalid for students from non-dominant cultures (e.g., Native Americans, African-American, Latinos, Asian-Americans) and argue that culturally biased tests contribute to inappropriate placements.

In this essay, many issues pertaining to equity and assessment are examined. It begins with a definition of culture and the implication of such a definition for understanding human behavior. Next, the philosophical underpinnings and research paradigms for studying human behavior are discussed. This is followed by a critical examination of the assumptions underlying standardized assessments and the challenges these pose for a nation committed to equity and excellence. The chapter ends with a number of recommendations for a more equitable assessment system.

DEFINING CULTURE

Culture is a socially constructed phenomenon that enables an understanding of the way of life of any social group. It is a multifaceted concept, the defining characteristics of which are many. As early as 1871, Taylor provided a definition of culture held by many anthropologists: "Culture or Civilization, taken in its wide ethnographic sense, is that complex whole which includes knowledge, belief, art, morals, law, custom, and other habits acquired by man as a member of society" (p. 1). Some eighty years later, a widely cited definition of culture in cross-cultural psychological research is provided by Berry (1976).

> .... We are born ignorant and helpless into a group. ... We proceed immediately to imitate and acquire these "group habits" of thought, feeling, and behavior; and the members of the group, at the same time, set about to indoctrinate us with those behavior patterns which they regard as right, proper, and natural."

Other investigators include values, language and a sense of continuity in their definitions of culture and distinguish between material and nonmaterial indices of it. For example, Geertz (1973) conceives of culture as

> "a historically transmitted pattern of meanings embodied in symbolic form by means of which men communicate, perpetuate and develop their knowledge about and attitudes toward life" (p. 89).

These definitions of culture emphasize the shared and learned ways of life of people that are passed down from generation to generation but there is another aspect of culture that includes structured relationships, which are reflected in institutions, social status, and ways of doing things. In an effort to synthesize these disparate definitions of culture, Gordon and Armour-Thomas (1991) distinguished five basic dimensions of culture:

1. the judgmental or normative dimension, indicative of the values and standards of a social group;
2. the cognitive dimension, which describes those categories of mentation such as attributions, social perceptions expressed through the language;

3. the affective dimension, which relates to the collective emotions of a social group, its common feelings and sources of motivation;
4. the skills dimensions describe the capabilities that members of a social group use in adapting to the social and economic demands of their environment;
5. the technological dimension describes the products or artifacts of a social group and includes the manner in which these are used.

CULTURE AND BEHAVIOR

Thus far, definitions of culture have emphasized those aspects by which the culture of a social group may be identified or characterized. But Kroeber and Kluckhohn (1952) pointed out that although cultural systems may be considered as products of action, their function as conditioning elements of further action should also be noted. The sense that culture influences human action suggests that culture is an explanatory concept, a functional phenomenon that enables an understanding and/or prediction of human behavior (Gordon, Miller and Rollock, 1991; Gordon and Armour-Thomas, 1991). Conceiving of culture as a functional or explanatory concept, we may seek answers to a number of questions of psychological significance, such as how do specific value systems of different social groups lead to different psychological outcomes? Do differences in norms for discourse between ethnic groups influence differential patterns of communicative competence? Do different child-rearing practices of boys within an Asian-American vs. a Native American community lead to differences in academic performance? Questions like these suggest that it is not enough to describe the values, language, or roles of members of a social group but, perhaps more important psychologically, it is necessary to examine the ways culture functions to socialize and shape group behavior.

CULTURAL DIVERSITY AND EQUITY

Differences in behavior as a function of cultural influences pose enormous challenges for any society such as the U.S., committed, at least in principle, to the ideals of equity and social justice. Are all cultural groups afforded equal access to the nation's resources to develop and demonstrate their talents and capabilities? In discussions of allocation of a society's resources, Gordon (1979) makes a distinction between equality and equity. For him, the concept of equality connotes sameness and the absence of discrimination whereas equity has more to do with distributional appropriateness and sufficiency. From this perspective Gordon argues that equal opportunity is not so much about providing all children with the same services, but about ensuring the appropriateness and sufficiency of treatment to the functional needs and characteristics of the persons being served. But Gordon and his colleagues (Gordon et al., 1991) recognized the difficulty in operationalizing the equity principle in a society where there is a tendency to make one's own cultural community the center of the universe and from this culturocentric perspective to view other cultural groups as deficient or inferior. In the subsequent paragraphs, we examine the philosophical issues associated with cultural diversity and equity and explore the research paradigm from which these issues have been studied.

PHILOSOPHICAL UNDERPINNINGS

Philosophically, adherence to the equity principle involves the right of diverse social groups to define and maintain their different ways of life and their obligation to have genuine mutual respect for each other's ways of life. What is at stake here is the coexistence of distinctive moral values, a subset of Berry's group habits of mind or Gordon's judgmental dimension of culture that some researchers consider the essence of cultural pluralism (Boyd, 1996; Cohen, 1993; Rawls, 1993). But the demonstration of democratic reciprocity is easier said than done for it requires more than token tolerance for cultural difference. Moon (1993) points out the challenge quite eloquently:

> moral pluralism does not simply involve the existence of what we might call "contingently" incompatible values—values that may come into conflict with each other depending upon circumstances. Rather it arises when different people resolve these conflicts in systematically different ways, or when they come to hold ends or principles that are inherently incompatible (p. 23)

Recognition of the equity principle implicitly embedded in the notion of cultural pluralism defined this way will pose enormous challenges for societies such as the United States, where historically, some ethnic groups (e.g., Native Americans, African-Americans, and Mexican-Americans) have endured varying conditions of domination or discrimination in the society. Boyd (1996) reminds us that moral commitment to the maintenance and promotion of cultural pluralism is threatening to those who are members of a culturally dominant group in the society.

In a related vein, the concept of "world view" offers further insight into issues pertaining to cultural diversity and equity. It refers to the "lens" through which a cultural group interprets reality as a function of cultural socialization (Ibrahim et al., 1994) and is based on a unique history of development of a cultural heritage (Dana, 1993). According to Dana (1993),

> The world view of a culture functions to make sense of life experiences that might otherwise be construed as chaotic, random, and meaningless. ... It is imposed by collective wisdom as a basis for sanctioned actions that enable survival and adaptation. (p. 91)

Observance of the equity principle would obligate members of diverse cultural groups to recognize each other's world views and to demonstrate behaviors consistent with genuine cross-cultural respect and tolerance. But as we try to show in the next section, much of the social science research referrable to groups from dominant and non-dominant cultures violates the equity principle when the researchers' lens leads to conclusions and interpretations that wittingly or unwittingly marginalize members of some non-dominant cultures.

RESEARCH PARADIGM

Increasingly, scholarly articles are appearing in mainstream journals that call attention to the implicit cultural bias among many researchers who study human behavior (Hilliard, 1996; Gordon, Miller and Rollock, 1990; Hall, 1997; Scheurich and Young, 1997). Consider a few of these titles: Coping with communicentric bias in knowledge production in the social sciences (Gordon et al., 1990); Coloring epistemologies: Are our research epistemologies racially biased (Scheurich and Young, 1997); the ethnocentric basis of social science knowledge production (Stanfield, 1985); Cultural malpractice: The growing obsolescence of psychology (Hall, 1997). A common position taken by these researchers is that the research paradigm reflects Western/Anglo/Euro epistemological traditions and there is a tendency to generalize findings to other groups that do not share those perspectives. Often, studies do not include operationally definable constructs of culture and when they do, terms like "culturally disadvantaged" or "cultural deprivation" betray an ethnocentric bias. Many years ago, Guthrie (1976) warned of the inherent danger of hegemonic research that seems to have been used to provide "empirical" evidence of the inadequacies of nonwhite male groups. Some twenty-five years later, we continue to wonder at the seeming lack of self-understanding among some researchers of the epistemological biases underlying their work. To the extent that findings from such research are used to guide the construction and administration of assessment procedures, the taint of ethnocentrism will more than likely permeate the entire assessment enterprise as well.

The linkage of research and assessment makes it easy to see how mistreatment or inappropriate educational placement may result from misdiagnosis through discriminatory assessment, the origins of which may be traced to erroneous generalizations and assumptions underlying culturally biased research conceptualization and methodology (see Gordon et al., 1990, and Hall, 1997, for a more comprehensive discussion of this issue).

THE CHALLENGE OF NONDISCRIMINATORY ASSESSMENT

Assessment is a process intended to elicit a sample of behavior from a set of tasks within a given domain in order to make judgments about an individual's probable behavior relative to that domain. Interpretations or judgments about behavior are oftentimes used to make decisions that have serious conse-quences for how and for whom the society's resources and opportunities are allocated. Genuine recognition and acknowledgment of cultural diversity and defense of standardized assessment create tension in a society committed to equity and social justice. On the one hand, respect for cultural diversity enti-tles members to develop and express behavior consistent with the values of their particular social group. On the other hand, though, acceptance of the standardization process in assessment implies the legitimacy of the values associated with those connected to the whole assessment technology: policy-makers, test designers and users. In a culturally diverse society, it is more than likely that some cultural groups share the values of the assessment con-stituency whereas others do not. The challenge for equity in assessment is to ensure that the judgments made about behavior of individuals and groups are accurate and that the decisions made do not intentionally or unintentionally favor some cultural group over another. This proposition may be difficult to operationalize for there are many culturally related factors relevant to the stan-dardized assessment process that could invalidate the information for some cultural groups. Consider some of these issues.

SUBJECT SAMPLING

A common practice in test construction is to include an adequate representation of subjects in the norming process. However, what constitutes adequate repre-sentation of some cultural groups remains problematic. For example, test con-structors often use census track data to operationally define socioeconomic sta-tus in their selection of subjects from Native American, African-American or Latino cultural groups. But within-group variations in social class do exist among these cultural groups, leading to differential exposure to teach-ing–learning experiences and, consequently, differential performance. Other demographic characteristics, such as ethnicity and language, are also confound-ed with culture, making attribution for differential performance among test-takers unclear. In other words, different cultural socialization experiences (beliefs, norms and values) of Latinos from Mexico, El Salvador, and Puerto Rico are more than likely to contribute to within-group variation in performance on academic, social or intellectual measures. There is little evidence to suggest that these issues are sufficiently understood among test designers in their efforts to select a representative sample of subjects.

BEHAVIOR SAMPLING

Another assumption of standardized assessment is that it measures what its designers claim it measures. More specifically, it assumes that the procedure measures the designer's conception of the construct of interest (e.g., language proficiency, intelligence, personality) and the behavior sampled is sufficiently represented in a sample of items. However, cultural groups may have conceptions or understandings of psychological constructs different from those represented in assessment measures. For example, conceptions of language proficiency vary. Some conceive of it as a composite construct with holistic qualities (Damico, 1991; Oller and Damico, 1991) whereas others view it as distinct bits and pieces of knowledge or specific abilities (Newmeyer, 1980). Consequently, inferences made about behavior on the basis of a particular conception of the construct will likely be valid for some groups but invalid for others. Ensuring sufficient representation of the construct in a sample of items will be meaningless for those children for whom the conceptualization of the construct is invalid.

EQUIVALENCE OF EXPERIENCES

An assumption regarding items that make up the assessment tasks is that such items are culturally fair in that they are not reflective of the experiences of one cultural group over another. But this assumption is invalid on a number of counts. First, there is tremendous variation in experiences within and between cultural groups, since constructs such as intelligence, communicative competence, language proficiency, and emotional well-being may have different meaning or significance. Second, some sociocultural experiences promote the development and nurturance of psychological processes in different ways. To the extent to which assessment practices elicit competencies developed within a particular cultural niche, members of a cultural group exposed to such socialization would have an experiential advantage. Some critics argue that designers of assessment procedures (e.g., personality and intellectual assessment) have not sufficiently addressed the question of cultural compatibility in the tasks selected for assessment (Butcher, 1982; Helms, 1992; Lonner, 1981). Among the major types of cultural compatible fallacies are:

  (a) contextual nonequivalence: whether the sociolinguistic factors such as norms of discourse are not familiar to all children tested;
  (b) conceptual nonequivalence: the extent to which task attributes (e.g., content of stimulus materials) do not have the same meaning for children from different cultural backgrounds;
  (c) linguistic nonequivalence: the extent to which the language used in standardized assessments does not have the same meaning for children from different cultural backgrounds.

THE ASSESSMENT CONTEXT

Another assumption of the assessment process is that all children understand the norms of discourse within the assessment context and therefore responses allow for a judgment of competence. However, the sociolinguistic patterns of some children reflect a style of communicating that may be different from the expectations of the standardized assessment setting, thus making it difficult to distinguish competence from communication style (Armour-Thomas, 1992; Miller-Jones, 1989). For example, Miller-Jones (1989) illustrated how the patterns of communication of an African-American child make it difficult to make accurate judgments of the child's intellectual functioning.

INTERPRETATION OF ASSESSMENT DATA

A basic tenet of the psychometric tradition in assessment is that the construct under consideration (e.g., intelligence, language, personality) can be assessed under uniform conditions in which all other factors are controlled. In this way, it is possible to observe and interpret behavior indicative of the particular construct of interest, irrespective of the cultural background or experiences of the examinee. Differences in test scores are usually reported according to race, social class and ethnicity categories. What is the point of contention, though, is the interpretation of score discrepancy in terms of deficits within either the person (genetic or biological inferiority) or the culture in which they are socialized (cultural deprivation). The dehumanizing and pejorative implications of deficit interpretations raise questions of whether any standardized measure could provide unbiased information with respect to culturally and linguistically diverse populations. Some critics point to the inadequate understanding of the role of culture and its influence on the development of constructs like intelligence (Rogoff and Chavajay, 1996), language (Harkness, 1986) and personality (Erikson, 1963). Others call attention to the ethnocentric research paradigms to prove the inadequacy of performance of members of cultural groups with subordinate status in the society (Stanfield, 1985; Jones, 1983). Yet others point to flaws in research methodology in using status characteristics, such as race or ethnicity, to classify members into groups without specification or measurement of these status characteristics (Helms, 1992; Betancourt, and Lopez, 1993; Phinney, 1996).

USE OF ASSESSMENT DATA

On the basis of assessment data, various kinds of psychoeducational decisions are made. Scores determine who gets tracked into low-level or honors classes, who is labeled gifted or mentally retarded, who gets placed in special education or in an English as a Second Language (ESL) class. There are two occasions when inequity may arise. The first arises to the extent that some cultural groups have greater opportunities in school to practice tasks similar to those used on assessment measures. For example, Rogoff and Chavajay (1996) describe the importance of formal schooling in enabling the development and nuturance of intellectual skills. The equity principle is also violated when opportunities for exposure to high-quality teaching and curricular offerings are differentially allocated. A number of researchers have noted that differences in academic achievement among groups can be explained by unequal access to high-quality curriculum and instruction (Darling-Hammond, 1994; Oakes, 1990).

TOWARD AN EQUITABLE ASSESSMENT SYSTEM

Assessment can be helpful when it enables decision-makers to plan and allocate resources commensurate with identified need. But it can also be used to reinforce or extend social inequities when it is used as an instrument for influencing the distribution of benefits and sanctions or in denying opportunities for optimal growth and development. As indicated in the previous section, judgments about behavior and decisions for subsequent services are not always accurate and decisions are not always made in the best interests of the test-takers. To enable the development and use of a more equitable assessment system, the following recommendations are made:

Extension of enabling resources and opportunities. An equitable assessment system is not likely to emerge unless policymakers make available certain institutional resources and conditions to enable the development of knowledge and skills *worth* assessing. This includes improving teacher capacity to teach children from culturally diverse backgrounds, providing underserved children exposure to high-quality curricula and other materials likely to enable the blossoming of the emerging potentials, and improving the capacity of mental health providers to work with clients from culturally diverse backgrounds. We share Gordon's (1995) and Madaus's (1992) view that equitable assessment measures cannot be produced until policymakers make available appropriate delivery standards (e.g., funding needed for educational and social resources) and support systems. We also support the National Council on Education Standards and Testing statement that a key condition for fair use of assessment results should be that schools ensure opportunity to learn, particularly for children who historically have been underserved in our schools.

Ownership in the assessment technology. Assessment may be considered "high-stakes" when the decisions have far-reaching consequences for its participants, consequences that may intentionally or unintentionally limit the quality of life for some cultural groups. Efforts to reduce inequity must involve the input of various groups likely to be adversely affected by the assessment technology. Staudenmaier (1989) has specified three technological constituencies wherein stakeholders may have a voice: *design constituency*—those with access to the necessary venture capital; *maintenance constituency*—those who will be benefit from the design and use of the technology; and *impact constituency*—those who will lose from the design and use of the technology. In conceiving of high-stakes assessment as a technology (e.g., Hanson, 1993; Madaus, 1992), all members of a society should have a right to be involved in technological choices that affect them (Winner, 1992). One way to realize that right is to ensure representation of key stakeholders at the design, maintenance and impact phases of the assessment process.

Genuine respect for multiple perspectives. Assessment of behavior is influenced by conception of the basic psychological process underlying behavior. However, conceptions of constructs such as intelligence, communicative competency, and literacy differ insofar as they embed meanings and values that shape the development and expression of behavior in particular ways for different cultural groups. Focusing on culturally mediated behavior in this way means that in a democratic society, the claims of others, or what Gordon calls multiple perspectives (1995), must be taken seriously. This means that to ensure equity in an assessment system, a genuine attempt should be made to understand and appreciate multiple perspectives regarding these constructs across the entire spectrum of the assessment process: design, maintenance and impact.

CONCLUSION

The role of assessment measures is to provide accurate information about an individual's or group's performance on a variety of tasks, and to make inferences about behavior on the basis of such evidence for a variety of purposes. In a culturally diverse society, committed to the principle of equity, the challenge for those connected to the assessment enterprise is to ensure accuracy of information and appropriateness of decisions for different groups in the society. In some sense, the dual recognition of cultural diversity and the standardization tenet of assessment create a dilemma that threatens to make the equity principle unenforceable. Rigid adherence to one is an implicit rejection of the other. We submit that efforts to resolve this seemingly intractable problem must broaden the representation of stakeholder groups across the entire assessment process. More importantly, though, social and economic changes in the larger society must ensure a common ground for all children. Unless all children are provided with equal opportunities to develop competencies, both before *and* after assessment, then tinkering with the psychometric properties of the measures themselves will do little to ensure non-discriminatory assessment.

CHAPTER 3

Ethical and Legal Issues in Cross-Cultural Assessment

Many professional organizations today, such as the American Psychological Association (APA) and the Council for Exceptional Children, have recognized that professionals who assess individuals from culturally diverse backgrounds must be trained to address the special needs of these populations if non-discriminatory assessment is to be provided (Gopaul-McNicol and Thomas-Presswood, 1998). The American Psychological Association (1993) stated that issues of culture do impact on the provision of appropriate psychological services. However, most training institutions still continue to exclude from their curricula courses addressing ethical and legal issues in cross-cultural assessment.

This chapter highlights the major court cases that forged new practices in the area of psychoeducational assessment and the provision of psychological services for clients from diverse cultural backgrounds.

CHANGES IN THE LEGISLATION AS A RESULT OF LITIGATION

Throughout the United States, public school education was built upon a segregational viewpoint that provided separate and unequal education to minority children. However, the National Association for the Advancement of Colored People (NAACP), encouraged by the increasing demand for accountability in psycho-educational assessment, has produced an emphasis on ethical concerns that expect competent behaviors on the part of professionals conducting the assessment. The result was an avalanche of significant court cases that shaped important social and educational laws throughout the United States. Most of the changes in the laws addressed several issues: (a) the administration and interpretation of tests by inadequately trained professionals; (b) making classification decisions based on the results of inappropriate tests; (c) provision of appropriate educational services; (d) stigmatization of students inappropriately placed in special education classes; and (e) involvement of parents in the assessment process (Gopaul-McNicol and Thomas-Presswood, 1998; Helton, Workman, and Matuszek, 1982).

Section 504 of the Rehabilitation Act – 1973: this civil rights law for individuals with disabilities established provisions relating to assessment (included in PL 94-142—that all disabled children have the right to free education) in the employment and educational settings.

The Family Education Rights and Privacy Act – 1974: this law stated that parents and all students 18 years of age or older had the right to examine all students' educational files or records, to object to any data in the files, and to indicate who can have and grant access to students' records. Parental consent was required before the district released any information in a student's file to other agencies (Wallace et al., 1982).

Carl D. Perkins Vocational Education Act – 1984: the intention of this law was to ensure that students who were disadvantaged or disabled were adequately served by vocational educational programs. It also emphasized that vocational planning and programming should be included in the Individual Educational Program, and the student with a disability must receive vocational assessment, counseling, and career development. Also, these students are entitled to special services, such as adaptation in curriculum, instruction, equipment, and facilities (Wallace et al., 1982).

Americans with Disabilities Act of 1990 (ADA): the purpose of this law was to safeguard the civil rights of individuals with disabilities in private employment and guarantee them access to all public services, public accommodations, transportation, and telecommunication.

Individual with Disabilities Education Act Amendments of 1995 (IDEA): this law was the third amendment made to PL 94–142. This reauthorization of PL 94–142 was intended to build on the basic purposes of the law (U.S. Department of Education, 1995). Each student must be ensured a free appropriate public education, determined on an individualized basis, designed to meet his or her specific needs in the least restrictive environment, protected through due process (U.S. Department of Education, 1995). This reauthorization focused on a number of key principles:

(1) Improve educational results for students with disabilities through higher expectations and access to the general curriculum.

(2) Address individual needs in the least restrictive environment.

(3) Provide families and teachers with the knowledge and training to effectively support students' learning.

In *Diana v. Board of Education* the plaintiff's contention was that inappropriate placement of Mexican American and Chinese students was based on discriminatory test results; this case established that testing be conducted in the student's primary language, the use of "nonverbal" tests, and the requirement to obtain extensive supporting data to justify special education placement (Kretschmer, 1991). Discriminatory testing procedures were also believed responsible for the inappropriate placement of Mexican-American and African-American students in EMR classes in the *Covarrubias v. San Diego Unified School District*; the court allowed a consent decree where plaintiffs could seek monetary damages for misclassification (Wallace et al., 1982); in addition, it recognized the need to provide informed consent prior to placement.

In 1974, the *Lau v. Nichols* case secured language programs necessary to provide equal educational opportunities. The court decision helped to foster guidelines now called the Lau Remedies, which focused on the identification of linguistically diverse students, assessment of their language proficiency and academic performance, and their placement in appropriate educational programs with bilingual instructional strategies (Kretschmer, 1991). The *Aspira of New York, Inc. v. Board of Education of the City of New York* case established the need to use proficiency tests to determine students' eligibility for a bilingual program.

The *Larry P. v. Riles* case has been called the "premier case involving bias in intelligence tests and placing children in programs for the mildly retarded" (Prasse and Reschly, 1986, p. 333). It was a class action suit filed in California on behalf of African-American students who had been inappropriately and disproportionately placed in EMR classes based on standardized IQ tests (Wallace et al., 1982). The decision was in favor of the plaintiff; it found that the school's methods of evaluating and placing students were inappropriate in two ways: standardized tests were determined to be discriminatory toward African-American children and the history of placement of African-American students in EMR classes pointed to unlawful, segregated intent (Prasse & Reschly, 1986). The use of standardized intelligence tests in California to place African-American students in EMR classes was prohibited. According to Prasse and Reschly (1986), to rectify these past practices, the court dictated extensive actions, including the following:

(1) Warning against the use of standardized tests on African-American students for identification as EMR and identification and placement in EMR classes.

(2) Requiring the use of nondiscriminatory and valid assessment instruments.

(3) Providing data to support the use of certain assessment instruments.

(4) Eliminating many African-American students from EMR classes.

(5) Reevaluating every African-American student previously identified as EMR without using standardized intelligence tests.

(6) Developing and implementing an IEP for every student found to have been misdiagnosed.

However, as McMillan and Meyers (1980) recognized, the injunction against the use of standardized intelligence tests had little effect on rectifying the disproprotionate percentage of culturally and linguistically diverse students placed in classes for the mentally retarded. Furthermore, McMillan and Meyers (1980) noted that: (1) to point to IQ tests as the prime culprit for the inordinate number of culturally and linguistically diverse students in EMR classes was to overlook the true complexity of overrepresentation; (2) school failure and not solely IQ tests were the primary determinants of EMR status; (3) instead of emphasizing why large numbers of culturally and linguistically diverse students were referred for assessment, the court focused on the issue of biased testing, and this prevented the development of effective educational assistance and instruction for this population of students; (4) the use of a quota system tɔ make sure that EMR population was representative of the general population of school-age children found opposition in many educators and scholars, including McMillan and Meyers (p.147); and (5) the fear of litigation made educators reluctant to place culturally and linguistically diverse students who really needed special education intervention.

The inappropriate placement of culturally and linguistically diverse students in EMR classes was not the only concern. *Lora v. New York City Public School Board (1977–1980, 1984)* shed light on the overrepresentation of African-American and Hispanic students in classes for students with severe emotional disabilities. The decision established: students must be assessed in their native language; assessment information must be gathered from a number of sources; parents must be informed of referral and of their due process rights; parents have the right to participate in evaluation and placement decision; and a structured observation of the student must be conducted by a member of the multidisciplinary team (Wallace et al., 1982). Finally, in *Dyrcia S. et al. v. Board of Education of the City of New York et al.,* the decision established the right to timely assessment and placement procedures. Bersoff (1981) concluded that there were there benefits from legal interference in assessment practices: (1) society had become more sensitive and aware of linguistic and cultural differences and the fact that testing may produce discriminatory results; (2) professionals had been made to confront and deal with the issue of accountability; and (3) the criticism leveled at standardized IQ tests has energized the field to develop improved and alternative means of evaluating cognitive abilities.

Many of these landmark cases generated court decisions that were translated into an amalgamation of federal dictates held in such Public School laws as 94–142 (i.e., the Individuals with Disabilities Education Act – IDEA – 1995). Six principles formed the core of this legislation:

FREE AND APPROPRIATE EDUCATION

This law guarantees a free and appropriate public education to all children with disabilities, regardless of the severity or nature of the disabling condition.

LEAST RESTRICTIVE ENVIRONMENT

Each child with a disability should be educated, whenever possible, in the least restrictive environment, with great emphasis on educating the student with his or her non-disabled peer.

Funding. The federal government was expected to provide to states the funding necessary to help insure the success of the law. However, the government never funded the law to the degree initially expected (Prasse, 1986).

NONDISCRIMINATORY ASSESSMENT

The law provides safeguards and guidelines to protect the rights of linguistically and culturally diverse students by dictating specific testing and placement procedures:

(1) A student must be assessed in his/her native language.

(2) Tests must evaluate what they were intended to evaluate (i.e., they must be valid).

(3) Assessors or test administrators must be appropriately trained to administer and interpret specific tests.

(4) Results yielded by the tests must be an accurate indication of a student's ability and achievement and not a reflection of sensory, manual, or speaking impairments, unless the test is designed to assess one of these domains (Wallace et al., 1982).

(5) Placement decisions cannot be made on the basis of any single factor. The decision must be made by a multidisciplinary team or group of educational practitioners.

(6) Student must be evaluated in all areas of suspected disability, which includes academic, achievement, motor ability, hearing, emotional, vision, social and emotional, and communicative skills.

(7) Every student identified as having a disabling condition must be reevaluated every three years by reviewing existing evaluation data regarding the student and focusing on the student's present level of performance and educational needs. The reevaluation must determine if the child continues to have the impairment and needs continual special education services.

(8) Initial evaluation should focus on instructional relevant information in addition to determining a disability.

INDIVIDUAL EDUCATIONAL PROGRAM (IEP)

Once the assessment has been conducted and the student is identified as having a disability, an IEP is developed based on criterion-referenced assessment rather than a norm-referenced test. The IEP is like a legal contract between the school district and the parent. It identifies the student's present level of performance or areas of strengths and weaknesses, and provides instructional objectives and goals to improve several areas of functioning, such as the student's academic, social-emotional, and management needs. The IEP is tailored to the specific needs of the student.

DUE PROCESS AND PARENTAL INVOLVEMENT

In order to ensure that parents have input into the assessment and placement processes, public agencies are expected to notify parents in writing when there has been a referral for assessment and to obtain the parents' written consent before conducting the assessment or placement. Parents also have the right to participate in the decision process for placement and can request an independent evaluation. The parents must be notified of their rights in writing and they must receive an explanation of the results of the assessment. Parents have the right to inspect the records or files and to disagree with any information contained in that file, and request an amendment. Finally, the school district is responsible for protecting the right to confidentiality of the student's records or files. Parents have the right to be made aware of who has access to their child's records and to request copies of the records.

ETHICAL ISSUES

Many organizations (e.g., American Psychological Association, National Association of School Psychologists (NASP)) have developed codes of ethical behavior standards that address the special needs of culturally and linguistically diverse populations. However, not all these organizations have incorporated them into their general set of ethical standards of conduct. The standards that have been developed address issues that pertain to assessment and treatment. In 1988, a Task Force was established by APA on the Delivery of Services to Ethnic Minority Populations in light of the increased awareness of psychological needs associated with ethnic and culturally diverse populations (APA, 1993). This Task Force developed a set of general principles that were intended to be suggestions for psychologists working with linguistically and culturally diverse children and families (APA, 1993). These sets of principles were titled the "Guidelines for Providers of Psychological Services to Ethnic, Linguistic, and Culturally Diverse Populations." Sue, Arredondo, and McDavis (1992) addressed the issue of cultural and linguistic diversity in the area of counseling in a paper published in *The Journal for Multicultural Counseling and Development*, and in the *Journal of Counseling and Development* titled "Multicultural Counseling Competencies and Standards." Both papers (APA's and Sue et al.'s) set forth recommended ethical practices. A review of these manuscripts yielded three major coordinating principles of concern: competency, intervention strategies, and respect for cultural differences. The following recommendations are made by APA (1993) and Sue et al. (1992) and were supported by Pedersen (1995), Ponterotto, Casas, Suzuki, and Alexander (1995), and Gopaul-McNicol and Thomas-Presswood (1998):

COMPETENCIES

(1) Psychologists should recognize the limits of their skills, training, and expertise in working with culturally and linguistically diverse children and families and should seek appropriate training, guidance, and consultation with experts or defer to other trained professionals.

(2) When assessing individuals from culturally and linguistically diverse backgrounds, psychologists must understand the limits of the assessment instrument or procedures (i.e., validity and reliability) with particular culturally and linguistically diverse groups. The resulting data should be interpreted in light of the cultural and language factors impacting on most assessment situations. The psychologist must understand how cultural and linguistic factors impact on the assessment process.

(3) If the client is bilingual or IEP, linguistic factors may present a barrier to the assessment or therapeutic situation. Consequently, the psychologist should interact in the primary or dominant language of the student. He or she must not only be able to understand the verbal messages but the nonverbal ones as well. If the psychologist is unable to do so, he or she must consider

either using an interpreter or referring the case to another professional competent in the language of the student or client.

(4) It is not sufficient just to understand how cultural and linguistic factors impact on the assessment and therapeutic process, but the psychologist must also document in the records cultural and sociopolitical factors.

RESPECT FOR CULTURAL DIFFERENCES

It is not sufficient for psychologists merely to understand that cultural differences do have an impact, but psychologists must also respect the fact that they exist. Respect allows psychologists to safeguard the rights of their students, to incorporate into their practice strategies that are sensitive to the cultural and linguistic needs of the student, and to recognize the limits of their skills and expertise. However, in order to understand and accept these differences, the psychologist must have an understanding of how their personal cultural and sociopolitical background and experiences impact on psychological processes.

INTERVENTION STRATEGIES

(1) Psychologists should understand how cultural, linguistic and religious practices influence the diagnosis and consider a differential diagnosis.

(2) Psychologists should understand the sociopolitical aspects of student life (e.g., discrimination, racism, poverty, immigration, and acculturation) as well as the client's world view, since it is the framework from which the student evaluates and sees society and him- or herself.

(4) Psychologists must remain up to date with the research as it pertains to working with culturally diverse individuals.

CONCLUSION

Today, practices in the areas of assessment, especially in the school setting, have been guided by legislation that emanated from court decisions intended to address issues of discriminatory assessment, lack of due process, and inappropriate placement of culturally diverse students in classes for the EMR or Emotionally Disabled children. Out of the many effort to rectify or correct traditional assessment practices which were discriminatory, PL 94-142 (the Education for All Handicapped Children Act) and the subsequent Individuals with Disabilities Education Act Amendment of 1995 were formed to safeguard the rights of all children and to guarantee a free and appropriate education.

Although several organizations have developed ethical standards for working with linguistically and culturally diverse children, the inclusion of these standards into their general set of ethical standards have been relatively slow (Gopaul-McNicol and Thomas-Presswood, 1998).

We close on a note from Korman (1974) who captures ethical concerns in the following statement:

> The provision of professional services to persons of culturally diverse backgrounds by persons not competent in understanding and providing professional services to such groups shall be considered unethical (p. 105).

CHAPTER 4

Toward a Bio-Cultural Perspective of Assessment

INTRODUCTION

Historically, standardized tests are designed to appraise differences in individual and group behavior for a given construct, such as language, intelligence, and personality. The general assumption is that under standardized conditions, in which other variables are controlled, cognitive, language, or personal functioning can become the focus of observation and interpretation. However, converging evidence from developmental research in a variety of areas of human functioning attests to the inseparability of culture and human development. Basically, the position, derived largely from the Vygotskian perspective, is that behavior, though rooted in some ways in biology, does not develop outside its sociohistorical context and cultural milieu (e.g., Bronfenbrenner, 1993; Gauvin, 1995; Rogoff and Chavajay, 1996; Super and Harkness, 1986). It follows from this perspective that assessment of behavior must take into account the cultural context and experiences within which biologically derived potentials develop and have meaning. The purpose of this chapter is twofold: (1) to discuss the basic tenets of a bio-cultural perspective and (2) to consider the implications of this view for assessment.

THE BIO-CULTURAL PERSPECTIVE

In our earlier work (Armour-Thomas and Gopaul-McNicol, 1998), we advanced the thesis of intelligence as a culturally dependent construct. In that work we argued that the human mind functions and develops within cultural niches, thereby making inevitable the co-mingling of biological and cultural processes. Although the range of cognitive potentials may be constrained by biological programming, these potentials are culturally channeled along different developmental pathways toward different endstates. Our review of theoretical and empirical literature on culture and human development has led us to make a similar claim about the cultural dependency of constructs such as personality and language. To be sure, as members of the species Homo sapiens, we are born with the capacities to acquire language and to develop intellectually and emotionally. However, when and how these biologically derived potentials grow and develop depends on the structure and organization of a cultural system to direct and regulate these biological potentials and enable their continuing transformation into higher-level psychological processes.

The inspiration for our position of the embeddedness of human development within a cultural system is derived from Vygotsky's sociohistorical theory that has generated a great deal of research since the publication of Mind in Society in 1978 in English. Although the focus of Vygotsky's work was in the area of cognitive development, it would appear that cultural forces shape and guide the development of language, cognition, and personality as well. We believe that various dimensions of human development are interdependent so that factors influencing one dimension are likely to influence other dimensions of the developing person. This conception of human development as an integrated whole implies that the process of cultural socialization is likely to influence the course and direction of language, emotional, and social development as well.

A fundamental assumption of the bio-cultural perspective is that characteristics of the person (e.g., language, personality, and cognition potentials) are reciprocally interactive with specific characteristics within the individual's culture. As human beings, we are born with capacities to acquire language, to think and feel in complex ways. However, selected attributes within a given culture determine when, how and under what conditions these potentials develop and are manifested in behavior. Similarly, the nature and quality of social interactions and other kinds of cultural stimulation determine how well our biologically derived capacities adapt to the ecologies in which we live and grow. The influence is therefore reciprocal or synergistic, in that the interplay within and between biological and cultural characteristics results in changes that become the basis for greater and progressively more complex development in both domains. (For a more comprehensive discussion of the interactionist perspective on human development, see Bronfenbrenner, 1993; Ceci, 1990; Gordon, 1984; Lewin, 1935; Murray, 1938). In our earlier work (Armour-Thomas and Gopaul-McNicol, 1998), we advanced a formulation for depicting the bio-cultural nature of these person-environmental interactions:

$$D_t \rightleftharpoons B_t = \int_{(t-p)} ST(PE)_{(t-p)}$$

B represents intelligence as cognitive behavior and lower-case *t* refers to the particular point at which it is observed; the symbol *f* stands for function and is used as an indicator for developmental processes through which conditions and attributes of the person and the environment are reciprocally interactive in ways that produce continuous change in cognition over time; lower-case *t-p* refers to the prior period when the reciprocal interactions between person and environment conditions and attributes were occurring to produce the cognitive behavior observed at the particular time of observation. *ST* refers to sustaining and threatening forces or conditions; *PE*, person and environmental factors. *D* refers to cognition as a developmental outcome observed at a particular point in time and the symbol $\rightleftharpoons$ is used to indicate that B_t and D_t can be used interchangeably.

In the section that follows, we describe two fundamental concepts of the bio-cultural perspective: *biologically derived characteristics and culturally dependent cognitions.*

BIOLOGICALLY DERIVED CHARACTERISTICS

The influence of biology on individual differences in behavioral development is well recognized in some areas of the field of psychology. Our review of the literature indicates that in all human beings, the genetic makeup, along with the dynamic organization and structure of the brain and nervous system, create biological predispositions for cognitive, emotional, and language development. Bronfenbrenner (1993) coined the term *developmentally instigative characteristics* to describe dispositions that induce or inhibit reactions from the environment in ways that affect subsequent psychological growth and development. Bronfenbrenner contends that these characteristics do not determine the course of human development but may be thought of as "putting a spin" on it. According to Bronfenbrenner, such characteristics

set in motion reciprocal processes of interpersonal interaction, often escalating
over time, that, in turn, can influence the course of development (p. 12).

Despite consensus about biological potentials associated with the construct
of personality, researchers have used various terms to describe an individual's
disposition toward environmental stimuli—situations, persons or events: *temperamental style* (Thomas and Chess, 1977; Gordon, 1988); *cognitive style*
(Messick, 1976); and *personal stimulus characteristics* (Bronfenbrenner, 1993).
It seems that some of these biologically based dispositions show a high degree
of stability and appear to be minimally responsive to environmental encounters, whereas others seem quite malleable and are reciprocally interactive with
particular aspects of the social and physical environment. Yet, there are other
response tendencies as Gordon (1988) calls them, that are motivational in
nature insofar as the individual exhibits initial interest and attention to certain
types of tasks and sustains a high energy level over the course of the activity
until goal attainment. Bronfenbrenner (1993) makes a similar claim in his use
of the concept of *selective responsivity* to describe the active orientation of a
person to be attracted by or demonstrate reaction to certain aspects of the
social and physical environment.

With respect to human cognition, Vygotsky identified a number of biologically derived characteristics (e.g., elementary perception, attention, and memory) as belonging to a lower class of psychological function. Similarly, Ceci
(1990) used the term *cognitive potentials* to define biologically based mental
operations with which all human beings are equipped at birth for encoding,
attending, scanning, transforming, and retrieving environmental input. How
these capacities develop and the nature and quality of their development are
due in no small measure to language.

There is some acknowledgement among researchers that language is, to a
certain degree, an innate human capacity, a medium through which we are
able to represent and make sense of our experiences in the world (Chomsky,
1956; Oller, 1989; Vygotsky, 1978). For example, Oller (1989) theorized
that, as human beings, we are born with a general semiotic capacity that may
be subdivided into three interrelated types of representational capacities:
sensory motor, kinesic and linguistic. Each one functions as a mediational
filter for different types of environmental stimuli that we encounter through
our five senses.

Although the research literature has provided some evidence for these
genetically based dispositions (Plomin, 1990; Henderson, 1982), there is a
growing recognition of the nonindependence of these human capacities from
the cultural processes that give them form and meaning. We turn now to a discussion of the defining attributes and mechanisms within the environment
that orchestrate the transformation of these biologically constrained potentials
into higher and more complex levels of psychological functioning.

DIMENSIONS OF CULTURE

In the previous chapter, we adopted a definition of culture the elements of which include the values, beliefs, and knowledge that are learned and shared by members of a social group. The fact that language is used as a vehicle through which members communicate with each other, and that it enables the acquisition of knowledge, skills and attitudes, makes it a key variable in the understanding of culture. Through our review of the literature from diverse disciplines (e.g., developmental psychology, education, psychology, sociolinguistics, and cognitive anthropology), we were able to discern at least three broad interrelated systems of culture that have psychological implications for the developing person: (1) value system; (2) symbol system; and (3) language system. A brief description of each follows.

VALUE SYSTEM

A value system consists of interrelated concepts that govern the day-to-day lives of a social group. These include values that define principles, attitudes and perceived obligations of a group as well as the norms that set the standards and expectations for their behaviors. It reflects Gordon's (1978) judgmental dimension of culture or Berry's (1976) group habit of mind—what people regard as right, proper, and natural. Beliefs are often implicitly understood and reflect a tacit consensus of assumptions about individuals and groups and their place within the society. Belief reflects a "mind set" that remains deeply entrenched in the psyche of a people despite the passage of time. The term is sometimes used interchangeably with "world view" or "ethos" that, according to Mbiti (1970), includes concepts such as understanding, attitude of mind, and perceptions that influence the way people think, act and speak in various situations of life. Collectively, we refer to these interrelated concepts as a *value system*, since it is likely that these concepts have their greatest impact as a cluster rather than a single entity. These intangible, yet powerful attributes of a culture provide structure, direction, and regulation for behavior. Through these functions, limits as well as opportunities are established for individual and group behavior, thereby enabling or constraining the course of human development.

SYMBOL SYSTEM

The symbol system describes the technologies (e.g., linguistic, pictorial, numerical, gestural) that enable the development and, ultimately, the expression of cognition within any given culture. It is through the use of a symbol system that the child acquires knowledge, the differentiation and elaboration of which enable him/her to make connections to events, objects, and persons within his/her environment. Some cultures use more than one symbol system so it is not uncommon that task demands reflect different permutations in content representation. For example, a task may require the processing of knowledge acquired through a dual modality of content: verbal-auditory; visual-spatialization; auditory-spatialization; pictorial-auditory; kinesthetic-auditory. Of course, even more complex permutations of these dual modalities may be represented in some tasks. A symbol system, like a value system, plays an enabling or constraining role in human development in that it inhibits or makes available options for learning. What is learned and how learning proceeds depends, in part, on the symbol system in which the task content is represented.

LANGUAGE SYSTEM

A language system describes a number of different ways in which a culture systematically communicates ideas, feelings, and thoughts through the use of words, sounds, gestures, or signals with commonly understood meanings. It shares with the symbol system the modality for communicating environmental stimuli. However, unlike the symbol system, the emphasis here is on the sociolinguistic conventions of a cultural group for organizing social interaction between an adult-child or peer collaborations.

These culturally valued media act as a vehicle for dynamic and mutual engagement in different kinds of tasks in the culture. A language system enables the acquisition of skills for organizing culturally valued knowledge and for communicating it to other members of the community. It also makes possible the acquisition and practice of culturally valued skills through the social interactions between significant other and child. Similar to the value and symbol systems, it plays a critical role in human development insofar as the nature and quality of learning is enabled or constrained by it.

In summary, we think that each culture has these subsystems and the story of human development is embedded within them. Although there is conceptual overlap among them, we believe that the collective impact on the child is greater than any one operating in isolation. How, then, do these interlocking cultural systems function to affect the psychological functioning of the child? We use two metaphors "cultural niche" and "learning experience" as a way to operationally seek an understanding of the psychological dynamics operating within and across the three cultural systems.

CONTEXT AS CULTURAL NICHES

We think that the concept of niche, first used in biological ecology, is a useful metaphor for understanding the context for human growth and development. Bronfenbrenner (1993) coined the term "ecological niches" to define those particular regions in the environment that are either favorable or unfavorable to the development of individuals with certain kinds of instigative personal characteristics. Super and Harkness (1986), Harkness (1990), and Gauvain (1995) used the concept of "developmental niche" to better understand the psychological processes of human development shaped by culture. When we use the concept of "cultural niches," we refer to those contexts within the larger environment wherein psychologically meaningful experiences occur for the developing person. Such contexts include the home, school, place of worship, community, peer group, or any other setting where opportunities exist for face-to-face social mediation of a culture's values, beliefs and attitudes to its members. While we consider these as the primary arenas for cultural socialization, there are other more distal or secondary settings within the larger society that may function as indirect contexts of cultural socialization. Parallel notions of multiple contexts of psychocultural influences are reported in the developmental literature (Bronfenbrenner, 1979, 1993; Gordon and-Armour-Thomas, 1991; Rogoff and Chavajay, 1996; Gauvain, 1995, Vygotsky, 1978).

EXPERIENCES WITHIN CULTURAL NICHES

We contend that it is within the cultural niche that biologically based dispositions are channeled along particular developmental trajectories through the process of cultural socialization. And it is through this process that biologically based dispositions in language, cognition, and personality are transformed over time into progressively higher classes of psychological functioning. Behavior observed at any point in time is thus a product of the synergistic influences of cultural and psychological processes operating between the person in interaction with forces within the cultural niche. The unit of analysis for understanding the interplay of biological and cultural phenomena is the nature and quality of the *learning experiences* to which the developing child is exposed. But what circumstances determine whether children will encounter the kinds of learning experiences critical for psychological growth and development?

The Laboratory of Comparative Human Cognition (1983) identified four ways by which culture creates regularities in children's environments in ways that support meaningful learning:

1. by arranging the occurrence or nonoccurrence of specific problem-solving environments;
2. by arranging the frequency of the same kinds of events in these learning environments;
3. by shaping the patterning or co-occurrence of events; and
4. by regulating the level of difficulty of the task.

For us, there are three defining attributes of experiences within any given cultural niche: (1) the persons (significant other/s and the child); (2) the tasks (the nature and level of complexity of the activity, its motivational allure, and the modality in which its content is represented); and (3) social mediation. Investigations of either person–process or person–task relationships may be subjected to manipulation as a way to better understand its unique influence on the behavior observed. However, these dyadic interactions should not obscure the fact that all three variables (person–process–task) interact in dynamic and complex ways to produce the behavior observed at any point in time.

PERSON–PROCESS

Social mediation describes the dynamic processes of mutual engagement that occur between adults, capable peers or any significant other and the child. It may be direct and involve face-to-face interactions or it may involve less direct social processes, as in apprenticeship situations wherein semi-structured opportunities are created for observational learning from experts as they demonstrate culturally valued skills in a given domain of interest.

Vygotsky (1978) provides some understanding for the mechanisms through which person–process interactions contribute to development, in this case, cognitive development. According to Vygotsky,

> Every function in the child's cultural development appears twice: first on the social level, and later on the individual level; first between people (interpsychological) and then inside the child (intrapsychological) (Vygotsky, 1978, p. 57).

At the first level, knowledge of a given culture is socially transmitted by adults and capable peers to children. Second, joint participation in the range of activities determined by the culture allows for the practice of certain skills and demonstration by adults or capable peers, so that children's current cognitive functioning may be strengthened or modified. Third, new cognitions are cultivated when the adult or capable peer shares in the responsibility for the task with the child. Assuming the role of an expert tutor, the adult models, corrects, clarifies, and explains concepts to the child in order that they attempt and complete the task according to the criteria established by the culture. Finally, the independent use of new cognitive abilities is encouraged when the adult or more capable peer works with the child on cognitively challenging tasks that they could not have successfully completed without guidance and support. Working with the child in his/her *zone of proximal development,* the adult models the task's appropriate behaviors, directs the child's attention to alternative procedures or approaches to the task, and encourages the child to try out his/her embryonic skills on some portion of the task. As the child's ability develops, the adult gradually reduces instructional support and allows him/her to assume greater independence in task solution. It is this type of *social scaffolding* that Vygotsky suggested as the mechanism for change in cognitive development. In analogous manner, we believe that the nature and quality of the relationship between significant other and child serve similar functions for the growth and development of language and personality.

PERSON–TASKS

The person–task concept is a useful one for understanding how individuals connect their existing cultural knowledge to new information of varying type and complexity. In addition, it clarifies the role of motivation in the acquisition of cultural knowledge and skills through active task engagement. An elaboration of these attributes follows.

Symbolic Representation of Information

Modes of representation are instantiations of a symbol system of a cultural group and include manipulatives, computers, maps, charts, various types of musical notation, written script, and forms of counting. Acquisition and mastery of knowledge depend, in part, upon the culturally sanctioned mode of representation within which information in tasks is encoded.

Vygotsky's (1978) conception of the symbolic feature of tool-mediated activity provides some understanding of its role in human development. Tools for Vygotsky are more than a collection of implements. Rather, they take on psychological significance when used to represent phenomena in collective human interactions. In his seminal work (1978, p. 127) he identified ancient tools, such as "tying knot"—used as a mnemonic device to facilitate retrieval. of information from memory; and "counting fingers"—used to support higher functioning that involved basic arithmetic operations.

Motivational Stimuli

An important characteristic of a task that is likely to influence performance is the extent to which it has properties that are likely to attract and sustain attention and emotional investment until its completion. Again, we look to the culture and ask the questions:

- What kinds of activities arouse individuals' attention and interest?
- What kinds of activities encourage them to sustain that effort with a level of intensity until task completion?
- And, perhaps equally important, what kinds of cultural practices support, maintain, and validate high levels of energy expenditure?

Answers to these questions have implications for human development for individuals are unlikely to engage and persist in progressively more complex activities unless there is the *will* to act. To the extent that the experiences have insufficient motivational pull, optimal learning may be constrained, which, in turn, may constrain optimal development. Conversely, experiences wherein the developing child sees relevance and value for himself or herself or decides that the goal is worth pursuing, then he/she is likely to engage in ways likely to facilitate learning and development.

Level of Complexity

Level of complexity refers to the cognitive difficulty of the task—both its form of representation and type and level of congnitive processing. Our reading of the empirical research suggests that knowledge and process are inextricably intertwined and, as such, behavior at any point in the child's development is likely to reflect the effects of a reciprocal interaction of knowledge representation and information processing.

Although the primacy of knowledge or processing remains unresolved in the literature, what is of interest to us is the notion that at a very early age, children seem predisposed to make sense of activities in which they are engaged and to construct schematic representations of environmental stimuli. Because of their inherent structure, these culturally coded knowledge structures are then used as interpretative frameworks for the acquisition of new knowledge.

Despite the lack of clarity with respect to the precise relationship between cognition and knowledge, we concur with the positions of Keil (1984), Chi (1978), and Ceci (1990), that the degree of elaboration and differentiation in the representation is perhaps the mechanism that makes possible the recognition of new relations and, consequently, the use of existing cognitive processes. And it is from this perspective that we speculate that the efficiency and accuracy with which some children respond to developmental tasks of increasing levels of difficulty may depend, in part, on the degree of elaboration and differentation of their knowledge structures.

IMPLICATIONS FOR ASSESSMENT

A fundamental purpose of assessment is to better understand human behavior: to consider performance on multiple tasks and in multiple contexts, to interpret performances and to use the data to make informed decisions about the individual or group. However, how these issues are addressed depends, in part, upon the assumptions from which the assessment designer and examiner operate. In the previous chapter, we identified a number of assumptions underlying standardized tests and the problems they pose for children whose cultural socialization is different from those of their peers in the mainstream culture. In this chapter, we have proposed a bio-cultural perspective of human development and believe that its assumptions pose different and additional questions for the assessment designer and examiner.

Earlier, we described two fundamental propositions of the bio-cultural perspective: the first one relates to the person–process–tasks interactions for an understanding of development or behavior. The second one has to do with the primary and secondary settings within and across which development unfolds or behavior is expressed. An obvious implication of this perspective is that the modality of the content, format, and context of assessment of psychological functioning should be, to some degree, compatible with cultural ways of knowing, feeling, and communicating. The questions for assessment are as follows:

1. Is the symbol system in which the competencies are represented familiar to the person being assessed?
2. Are there alternative symbol systems for assessing the competencies of interest?
3. Is the value system implicit in the competencies shared by the person assessed?
4. Is the language system used to communicate the competencies familiar to the person assessed?
5. Are there alternative language systems for assessing the competencies of interest?
6. Is the level of complexity in the competencies assessed commensurate with the prior knowledge of the person assessed?
7. Are there motivational factors within the primary settings likely to enhance or hinder performance on the competencies assessed?
8. Are there opportunities for assessing the competencies of interest in more than one primary setting?
9. Are there factors operating within the primary settings that can inhibit or promote performance on the competencies assessed?
10. Are there factors operating in more distal or secondary settings that can inhibit or promote performance on the competencies assessed?

11. Is the format in which the competencies are embedded familiar to the person assessed?

A BIO-CULTURAL ASSESSMENT SYSTEM

It is unreasonable to expect that any one measure would provide satisfactory answers to the questions consistent with a bio-cultural perspective of human development. Rather, an assessment system comprising both quantitative and qualitative measures is likely to provide comprehensive information on the developing person's psychological functioning. Some questions lend themselves to direct observation of the child in one or more primary setting. Others may require a clinical interview with the child and significant others in the child's life. Yet others may require self-reports, surveys, or questionnaires. These multiple forms of assessment are in line with Kaufman's (1979) hypothesis-testing approach where the role of the examiner in psychoeducational assessment is to "test" various hypotheses about the developing person's competence using multiple sources of data. In our previous work on intellectual assessment (Armour-Thomas and Gopaul-McNicol, 1998), a four-tier assessment system was proposed that we think has applicability to other areas of psychological functioning. The components of the multi-level assessment system are as follows:

PSYCHOMETRIC ASSESSMENT

Psychometric assessment describes any standardized measure of psychological functioning used to identify the individual's current level of performance. The purpose of this first tier of assessment is to locate individual strengths and weaknesses in any given domain of interest elicited under standardized conditions in a particular context.

PSYCHOMETRIC POTENTIAL ASSESSMENT

This procedure consists of any number of diagnostic probes within the standardized testing context, the purpose of which is to identify potentials that standardized measures by design are not likely to unmask. These strategies are particularly useful for children whose primary cultural socialization is different from those on whom the standardized test is normed. They provide value-added information about nascent potentials not yet fully developed or competencies not likely to be demonstrated under standardized testing conditions.

ECOLOGICAL ASSESSMENT

Ecological assessment consists of a series of informal procedures used to gather information about the behavior of the individual from direct observation in the contexts in which he/she functions. In addition, more indirect qualitative information may be derived through surveys, questionnaires or structured interviews with others who may have knowledge about the individual's performance in non-standardized settings.

OTHER INTELLIGENCES ASSESSMENT

This measure specific to intellectual functioning seeks information about the individual's other cognitive strengths beyond the realm of IQ testing. Adapted from Howard Gardner's work on multiple intelligences, the examiner asks a number of questions of the individual, his/her teachers, parents, coaches, or any significant others about the individual's bodily-kinesthetic, musical, and interpersonal competencies.

CONCLUSION

The bio-cultural perspective proposes that human behavior is a product that emerges from experiences within and across multiple settings. Critical attributes of experiences unfold across three overlapping subsystems: the value system, the symbol system and the language system, each of which has psychological implications for the developing person. More specifically, these experiences describe the synergistic interactions between characteristics of the developing person (biologically based dispositions) and tasks and significant other/s within cultural niches. Behavior observed at any point in time reflects these person–environmental interactions and, in this sense, it may be regarded as a bio-cultural phenomenon. In drawing implications for assessment, the perspective poses new and additional questions for the psychoeducational examiner. An assessment system comprising both quantitative and qualitative measures is recommended as a complement to standardized tests.

PART II

Practical Issues in Cross-Cultural Assessment

Assessing the Intellectual Functioning of Children from Culturally Diverse Backgrounds

Unlike those of other reform movements in U.S. education, educational goals in the 1990s are centered around the three E's: economics, excellence and equity. The prosperity of the nation is perceived as dependent on the capacity of schools to produce workers with deep conceptual understanding in various domains of knowledge and demonstrations of advanced skills of reasoning, problem-solving, and higher-order thinking. While concern for equality of educational opportunity is not a new concept in U.S. education, it is new to envision academic excellence for *all* children, irrespective of race, class, ethnicity, gender, and language or any other dimension of human diversity by which individuals and groups are categorized in the society. This vision of education for the nation's children suggests that assessments should identify individuals who are likely to succeed in educational opportunities and those who are at risk of failure or underachievement. Moreover, to ensure that the best education is availble to every student, assessments must inform and guide the implementation of educational experiences adaptive to the differential strengths and needs of all students. Traditional standardized tests of intelligence measure the kinds of knowledge and cognitive skills that are, in some respects, similar to those measured by standardized tests of academic achievement and do predict academic success for many students. As such, measures of intelligence should be considered in any assessment battery for educational purposes. Mindful of the criticisms of such measures for students from racial and ethnic minority populations (Armour-Thomas, 1992a; Armour-Thomas and Gopaul-McNicol, 1998; Cummins, 1991; Gopaul-McNicol, 1992a; Hilliard, 1996; Samuda et al., 1989; Williams, 1970) though, caution is urged in how and under what conditions standardized tests of intelligence are to be used in the educational arena.

Implicit in the use of standardized intelligence test data for these purposes is a notion that differences in test scores reflect fundamental differences in intellectual capacities and that the goal of assessment is to objectively sort children according to these underlying differences. Once accurately sorted, educational programs can be more readily matched to these underlying differences. The scientific legitimacy of this notion, however, is in serious question when judgments about intellectual capacity parallel race, class, and language differences, as is the legitimacy of educational placements. For example, it is a well-documented finding that the average performance of children from African descent differs by as much as one standard deviation on any standardized test of intelligence. It is also common knowledge that racial and ethnic minorities judged as "low ability" are placed in low-tracked and remedial classes or in special education programs (Persell, 1977; Slavin, 1987). But what exactly the differences in IQ scores mean and what the origins of such variations are have been controversial questions since Jensen's (1969) declaration that the differences are real and substantial—a sentiment echoed in Herrnstein and Murray's more recent book, *The Bell Curve* (1994).

The purpose of this chapter is threefold: (1) to examine the cognitive processes underlying standardized tests of intelligence; (2) to identify the difficulties that assumptions of standardized IQ tests pose for children of low-income, race/ethnic and linguistic backgrounds; and (3) to critically examine some promising alternatives to standardized tests of intelligence with a view toward a new direction for intellectual assessment.

STANDARDIZED TESTS OF INTELLIGENCE

Traditional tests of intelligence, often dubbed psychometric measures of IQ, are designed to tap mental abilities, many of which have been identified at various hierarchical levels. Usually, factor analytic techniques are used to examine a matrix of intercorrelations or covariances for a set of scores to uncover common patterns of individual differences in performance. The observed patterns or factors sometimes referred to as latent traits are presumed to be manifestations of individual differences in cognitive abilities as hypothesized by the theorist. Successive factorization of correlation matrices yields different numbers of factors at varying levels of generality. Spearman's (1927) two-factor theory, Thurstone's (1938) seven-factor theory, Horn's (1991) nine broad abilities, and Carroll's (1993) three-stratum theory are well-documented examples of the application of psychometric methodologies to infer the structure or organization of the human intellect. Many tests of intelligence are rooted in this psychometric conception and continue to be used as valid measures for sorting children according to these underlying factors or mental abilities. Although current IQ tests (e.g., The Wechsler scales, the Kaufman Assessment Battery, Binet: 4, and McCarthy scales, The Woodcock-Johnson Tests of Cognitive Ability–Revised) may differ in the number, type, or level of general abilities measured, they all include tasks of knowledge, reasoning, memory, and speed. Many of these tasks are embodied in verbal, spatial and quantitative content and some involve visual and auditory processing. Some test items reflect learning experiences that are similar to the learning experiences common in some home and school contexts. Consequently, it is not surprising that for some children, IQ tests accurately predict grades and scores on achievement tests.

Despite the consistent findings in the literature regarding the reliability and validity of IQ tests, some critics have registered concerns about their usefulness in educational decision-making for children from diverse backgrounds. For example, Glaser (1977) claimed that such tests give go/no-go selective decisions but do not provide information that is sufficiently diagnostic for the conduct of instruction. Gordon (1977) made a similar point when he argued that, at best, test data analysis provide gross characterization of success and failure of students in relation to some reference group but such analysis provides little information about the process by which individuals engage the task, and is insensitive to an individual's differential response tendencies. But as Gordon asserted, the description of these characteristics of behavioral individuality is of crucial importance in the design and management of teaching and learning transactions. These concerns have particular relevance for some racial and ethnic minority populations who, as groups, have consistently performed poorly on standardized tests of academic achievement relative to their Euro American peers. Others question the validity of IQ test scores for many racial and ethnic minority children and youth (Armour-Thomas, 1992b; Armour-Thomas and Gopaul-McNicol, 1998; Cummins, 1984, Gopaul-McNicol, 1992, 1991; Lipsky and Gartner, 1996; Samuda, 1975; Samuda, Kong, Cummins, Pascual-Leone and Lewis, 1989; Williams, 1970). In the next section, we summarize some of the more persistent claims of bias critics have made against the use and interpretation of results of standardized IQ tests for racial and ethnic minorities.

CONCERNS ABOUT STANDARDIZED TESTS OF INTELLIGENCE

Generally, proponents of standardized measures of intelligence justify the comparison made about intellectual performance between different cultural groups on the grounds that such measures meet at least four implicit criteria: (a) the tasks as constructed are culturally fair—that is, items do not favor any particular cultural group; (b) the tasks assess the cognitive abilities underlying intellectual behavior; (c) the tasks could sufficiently elicit the deployment of particular mental operations; and (d) accurate interpretations could be made from comparing the average IQ scores of different cultural groups. When these criteria are applied in the assessment of intellectual functioning of children from certain racial and ethnic groups, numerous difficulties arise that raise serious questions about the validity of comparative judgments about their performance. Consider some problems of standardized tests for these populations:

ITEM SELECTION BIAS

Any intelligence test construction procedure involves the standardization of the test on a representative sample. This means, in the case of the U.S. society, the majority of subjects will come from the dominant group—Anglo or European-Americans. A minority of groups will make up the rest of the sample—groups of non-European origin, including Native Americans, African-Americans, Mexican-Americans, Caribbean-Americans, Asian-Americans, and Pacific Islander-Americans. During the early stage of item development, the majority of items selected for try-out will obviously reflect, to some extent, the prior learning experiences of the Anglo or European-American group. Since academic achievement correlates with any standardized test of intelligence, this means that the learning experiences are similar to those acquired through formal schooling.

It cannot be assumed that the learning experiences of the majority group are similar to those of the minority groups (e.g., Boykin, 1986; Ogbu, 1986). Nor can it be assumed that the learning experiences derived from schooling for majority children are similar to those of minority groups, particularly those from low-income backgrounds (Oakes, 1990). Even if items reflective of the prior learning experiences of minority groups were included in the early phase of item development, they would more than likely be screened out during item analysis. A common psychometric practice in test construction is to retain only those items that correlate with the total test and that are of moderate difficulty. Items that are appropriate for minority groups, more often than not, will be difficult for the majority group and will not correlate well with the total test (e.g.,

Williams' (1975) BITCH 100 (Black Intelligence Test of Cultural Homogeneity)). Thus, the process of item selection for an intelligence test does involve some bias against minority groups. (See Cummins, 1984, for a more comprehensive discussion of these issues pertaining to item selection bias.)

LACK OF SPECIFICITY ABOUT COGNITIVE PROCESSES

Although psychometric studies of cognitive abilities have identified a number of cognitive processes that underlie performance on intellectual tasks (e.g. Carroll, 1993; Horn, 1991) there is no consensus about how many and which processes combine to produce behavior indicative of intelligence. Horn (1993) in describing the difficulty of identifying with precision these processes remarked

> specifying different features of cognition is like slicing smoke - dividing a con tinuous, homogeneous, irregular mass of grey into ... what? (p. 198).

Lack of specificity of cognitive processes when describing intellectual behavior in assessment situations is likely to favor some cultural groups but hinder others. Three decades ago, Messick and Anderson (1970) called attention to the fact that these same tests may measure different processes in minority children from low income backgrounds than it measures white middle class children. A similar concern was articulated by Farnham-Diggory (1970 who suggested that the multiplicity of cognitive processes in Thurstone's Primary Abilities Test (PMA) made it difficult to determine which of these processes pose difficulties for children of African heritage. In our own work, it was not always clear when children from culturally and linguistically diverse backgrounds answered items incorrectly, that these errors were due to inaccurate or inefficient deployment of cognitive processes or to unfamiliarity of the content of the test items.

CONTENT BIAS

When comparisons are made between cultural groups on standardized measures of intelligence, inaccurate assumptions about aspects of the task requiring the deployment of mental processes may be made. In other words, differences in cognitive processes may be a function of variability in dimensions of tasks within a particular cultural context. Many cross-cultural studies have reported that the familiarity or unfamiliarity of content may constrain or promote the efficient or accurate elicitation of cognitive processes in tasks involving memory, reasoning, perception and problem solving (e.g. Lave, 1977; the Laboratory of Comparative Human Cognition [LCHC] 1982). In these studies, researchers focused on the domain-specific thinking of people as they solve problems routinely encountered in their culture. For example, in an early cross-cultural study, Gay and Cole, (1967) assessed classification competencies between school and unschooled Liberians and U.S. schooled children by using tasks involving culturally appropriate content: bowls of rice and geometric blocks. African subjects were able to perform as competently when the tasks involved rice as the stimulus as did their U.S. counterparts who used geometric shapes. In contrast, decrements in performance were observed for both groups when the content of the stimulus materials were reversed. In other words, African children classified geometric shapes as poorly as did the U.S. children sorted rice. More recently, several researchers use concepts like everyday cognition (e.g. Rogoff and Chavajay, 1995) and practical intelligence (Neisser, 1979, Sternberg, 1985, Sternberg and Wagner, 1986) to better understand the thinking competencies of individuals and groups underlying their performance on culturally-familiar tasks in their own communities.

The LCHC (1982) used the concept of "functional stimulus equivalence" to account for these content-specific findings. This suggests that in order to make valid comparisons of intellectual performance between cultural groups, it is critical that the stimulus attributes of the task are equivalent for both groups in its ability to elicit the cognitive processes under investigation. From our experiences with standardized tests of intelligence with children from culturally diverse backgrounds, it does not appear that test designers have sufficiently addressed the issue of functional equivalence in item construction or selection.

UNFAMILIAR SOCIOLINGUISTICS

One of the hallmarks of intelligence testing is the adherence to standardized procedures during its administration. One aspect of these procedures has to do with examiner-examinee interactions. When to probe for more information, how to respond to the examinee's queries, how much feedback to give- are all governed by a strict protocol using a standard format. However, such constraints of the testing environment may preclude an accurate estimation of intellectual competence of some children from culturally diverse backgrounds. An example of this problem concerns the dynamics of sociolinguistics among ethnic minority children from low income backgrounds. Sociolinguistic variables are courtesies that govern verbal interactions that can have a positive or negative impact on student motivation to engage in a task or not. Miller-Jones (1989) provided some excellent examples of the verbal interactions between an examiner and an African- American child to demonstrate how such interactions of the testing context may result in erroneous judgments about the intellectual functioning of that child. The question and response exchange clearly indicated that the child did not understand or was not familiar with the social dynamics within the testing context. In short, in a standardized testing context, the norms of discourse are predetermined and performance differences could result to the extent that children's sociolinguistic patterns of communication are different from the examiner's script.

Test Interpretation Bias

Comparisons of intelligence test scores on the basis of ethnic classification are likely to lead to bias in interpretation since there is considerable heterogeneity within such groups in terms of family structure, geographical region, gender, socioeconomic status, language, educational orientation and perceived discrimination. For example, Phinney (1996) identified at least three aspects of ethnicity for ethnic groups of color in the United States (e.g., Native Americans, African-Americans, Latinos, Asians, and Pacific Islanders) that may have psychological relevance for influencing behavior:

- the cultural values, attitudes, and behaviors that differentiate ethnic/racial groups;
- identity—the perception of what it means to the individual to belong to an ethnic/racial group;
- the experiences associated with minority status in the U.S. (e.g., discrimination, prejudice, and a sense of powerlessness)

These features of psychological characteristics are similar to those identified by Sue (1991), who, like Phinney (1996), views them as overlapping and confounded constructs. Thus, an ethnic label alone is not enough to interpret differences in performance between ethnic groups. To understand intellectual behavior would require an unpackaging of the multiple psychological processes associated with the label, as a number of researchers have recommended (Betancourt and Lopez, 1993; Phinney, 1996; Poortinga, van de Vijver, Joe, and van de Koppel, 1987; Whiting, 1976).

One of the methodological difficulties associated with the unpackaging of psychological processes, however, is that researchers and pollsters may not have fully understood or appreciated their importance in influencing behavior. As Betancourt and Lopez (1993) noted, research instruments and surveys often require subjects to indicate race by selecting among confounded status variables (White, Black, Latino, Native American, Asian). Zuckerman (1990) cautioned that the loose way in which race, culture, and ethnicity are treated may contribute to interpretations of findings of observed differences among groups that reinforce racist conceptions of human behavior.

Even in cases where researchers try to minimize the confounding of status characteristics, it is not clear that they succeed. For example, in statistically controlling for the effects of socioeconomic status among Latino or Asian children in a study of, say, intelligent behavior, a researcher can unwittingly mask the effects of language and culture. To the extent that these two latter characteristics are differentially experienced by members who are located in different class positions, one can misattribute to socioeconomic status, the influence of language or culture or both.

Comparisons of average IQ test scores of Black and White children are equally problematic when using the race label to make group classifications. As Helms (1992) noted, tremendous variation may exist within Black and White populations because of:

(a) voluntary and involuntary interracial procreation

(b) the tendency of researchers to assign subjects to one group or another on the basis of physical appearance

(c) the decision of some visible racial or ethnic groups who appear White to disappear into White society (a process called "passing" in Black culture)

(d) the possibility that immigrants who would be considered Black if they were born of similar parentage in this country classify themselves as White or other than Black (p. 1085).

Variations in perceptions of race also exist in other countries. In a recent review of conceptions of race as a socially constructed phenomenon, Eberhardt and Randall (1997) described the fluid continuum by which race is defined in Brazil, Latin America and Caribbean countries. Factors such as economic and geographic mobility are allowed along the continuum, as are a wide range of colors. In Caribbean and Latin American countries, it is not uncommon for individuals to change color or to have different perceptions of physical attributes such as hair texture and skin pigmentation as a function of economic mobility. According to these researchers, in these countries, money "whitens." Thus, an interpretation of differences of IQ scores between subjects of European and African descent on the basis of racial categorization is indefensible.

TOWARD NONDISCRIMINATORY PRACTICES IN INTELLECTUAL ASSESSMENT

Despite the claims of bias in standardized tests of intelligence, we contend that these measures can be used for educational purposes if accommodations are made to enhance the instrument's validity for racial and ethnic minorities and if other measures are used in conjunction with them. These validity enhancement procedures would need to:

- be sufficiently diagnostic so as to uncover emerging cognitive potentials that the standardized IQ tests were not designed to measure but which are relevant for academic performance and achievement;
- ascertain the examine's level of acculturation prior to IQ testing;
- ascertain the probable contribution of other context factors that may be used to facilitate a more valid interpretation of scores obtained on the standardized IQ measure.

However, before seeking this information, some effort must be made to rule out factors that may be responsible for the examinee's problems. A discussion of these issues follows.

PREASSESSMENT ACTIVITIES

Prior to the administration of any measure to assess intelligence, a differential diagnosis should be conducted to ascertain factors that may influence the examinee's performance during the test administration. The examiner would need to review the examinee's school records and interview or administer a questionnaire to a parent or significant other in the examinee's life to obtain information on questions such as:

- Does the examinee have any ailments that may impede his/her functioning during the administration of the test?
- Is the examinee proficient in the English language?
- Are the examinee's prior educational experiences (learning style, interrupted schooling, test-taking experiences) likely to influence his/her performance on the IQ measure?
- Are there factors in the examinee's culture (e.g., conception of time, familiarity of test content, response style) that may influence performance on the test?
- Are there factors at home (e.g., recency of arrival in the U.S., literacy level, educational values) that may influence the examinee's motivation during the testing situation?

PSYCHOMETRIC ASSESSMENT OF INTELLIGENCE

Any standardized measure of intelligence may be used to ascertain a manifest or actual level of intellectual functioning. This measure will yield information on the strengths and weakness of the examinee's developed intellectual ability on decontextualized verbal and nonverbal tasks in a contrived testing environment. These tasks require the examinees to show their knowledge and skills in areas such as reasoning, memory, visual-spatial organization, vocabulary, comprehension, problem-solving, and speed of processing. As indicated earlier, it is important to gauge these intellectual competencies since, to some extent, they underline performance on standardized achievement tests.

ASSESSMENT OF COGNITIVE POTENTIALS

As indicated earlier, critics of IQ tests argue that some children from racially and ethnically diverse backgrounds have not had learning experiences comparable to the majority of their peers who have been socialized in the mainstream culture of the U.S. Consequently, they perform poorly on IQ measures that erroneously assume equivalent experiences. To obtain a more accurate picture of their true abilities, modifications must be made in the administration of any standardized IQ test. Dynamic assessments (Samuda et. al., 1989; Feuerstein, 1979; Lidz, 1987), as these accommodations within the testing situation are called, go beyond standardized instructions to probe for nascent cognitive abilities. These clinically derived results are then used, in conjunction with psychometric test scores, to make more valid interpretations of the examinee's performance. These dynamic assessments include elimination of time limits, test-teach-test procedures, use of additional probes, cues, and scaffolding techniques. Each is elaborated upon below.

The Learning Propensity (formerly, Potential) Assessment Device

This instrument is based on the theory of structural cognitive modifiability and on mediated learning experience that holds that (a) human beings have a unique propensity to change their cognitive functioning in response to changing demands of life experiences and situations that they encounter; and (b) change in cognitive functioning is facilitated through a mediated learning experience that involves the intentional actions of a person to interpret, select, elaborate, and filter what has been experienced (Feuerstein, 1979; Feuerstein, Falik, & Feuerstein, 1998). Unlike conventional IQ measures, with the emphasis on ascertaining what an individual is able to do at a given moment in time, the focus here is on what the individual can become able to do, in both present and future interactions. Several instruments make up the LPAD battery, a series of testing-in-the-act-of-learning procedures. They permit the examiner to observe the examinee's response to tasks and use this information to stimulate and elicit changes in performance of the examinee. In a recent discussion of the LPAD process of dynamic assessment, the authors (Feuerstein et al., 1998) identified the kinds of diagnostic data that may be gathered by using these instruments:

- The readiness of the examinee to grasp the principle underlying the initial problem and to solve the problem
- The amount and nature of investment required in order to teach the examinee the given principle
- The extent to which the newly acquired principle is successfully applied in solving the problems that become progressively more different from the initial task
- The differential preferences of the examinee for one or another of the various modalities of presentation of a given problem
- The differential effects of different training strategies offered to the examinee in the remediation of functioning, involving the criteria of novelty, complexity, language of presentation, and types of mental operation (pp. 120–130).

Psychometric Potential Assessment

This measure is the second tier in Armour-Thomas and Gopaul Mc-Nicol's (1998) bio-cultural approach to intellectual assessment. It consists of four strategies that may be used in conjunction with any psychometric measure of intelligence. Collectively, these probes are intended to provide supplementary information on the cognitive functioning of the examinee that goes beyond what is provided by the conventional standardized measure of intelligence for children and youth. It was developed on the basis of our experiences using the Wechsler Intelligence Scale for Children–III with children from culturally and linguistically diverse backgrounds (U.S.-born African-American and Latinos, and children of color from the United Kingdom, English- and Spanish-speaking Caribbean).

Clinical observation of children during the standardized administration of the WISC-III showed that they approached timed tasks in a deliberate and slow manner, in spite of instructions to "work as quickly as you can." They seemed totally lost when asked to work with items on the nonverbal subtests (e.g., Block Design and Object Assembly), even after the standardization instructions were provided by the examiner. Many of them remained silent or shrugged their shoulders when asked to define words. Others appeared frustrated on the Arithmetic subtests with protestations of "I can't do this in my head."

Post-observation interviews with children and permission from their families to readminister some items on the WISC-III with modifications corroborated our clinical observations that the IQ measure did indeed underestimate the cognitive capacities of many of them. Their performance improved when they were allowed to work at their own pace. When given the opportunity to use paper and pencil, they often solved the arthmetic problems. They demonstrated understanding of words when allowed to say them in sentences and some of them showed dramatic changes in their performance when they were taught and retested on nonverbal items.

On the basis of these experiences, we developed four procedures that are likely to uncover hidden cognitive potentials of children. Although initially designed for use with the Wechsler Intelligence Scale for Children III, these probes can be used in conjunction with any psychometric test of intelligence that involves speed, mental problem-solving, decontextualized vocabulary, and manipulation of nonverbal stimuli. A description of each procedure follows:

a. *Suspending time.* After the subtest has been administered in accordance with standardized instructions, the examiner allows the examine to complete the item at his or her own pace.

b. *Contextualization.* After the administration of the vocabulary items in the standardized fashion, the examiner can ask examinees to contextualize the words in sentences. For example, the examiner can say to the examinee. "Please say the word _____ in a sentence."

c. *Paper and pencil.* After the standardized administration of the arithmetic items, the examiner can say to the examinee who fails the problem-solving items, "Please use this paper and pencil and try to solve the problem."

d. *Test–Teach–Retest.* Following the standardized administration of the nonverbal items (Block Design, Picture Arrangement, or Object Assembly and failure after trials, the examiner teaches and retests the examinee. In teaching, the examiner may explain the meaning and purpose of the task, give feedback on examinee's responses, probe for misunderstandings and encourage task completion.

Assessment of Context Variables

There are many contextual factors that may affect the validity of IQ scores for children from culturally diverse backgrounds, such as differential socialization and educational experiences, level of acculturation, or sociodemographic classifications. In the psychological literature, these variables are called moderator variables (Dana, 1993; Lewis, 1998; Saunders, 1956). The purpose of using them, as Dana (1993) reminds us, is to

> prevent genuine differences from being ignored, disregarded, or minimized, while still being able to employ measures that have been designed for and standardized on Anglo-Americans (p. 115).

Thus, assessment of these moderator variables should go hand in hand with the administration of any psychometric measure to: (a) ascertain the extent to which an examinee's performance is affected by them and (b) use the data obtained in the interpretation of performance of children from cultures different from the one on which the psychometric IQ test was normed. Structured interviews, questionnaires, and behavioral observation are commonly used to gather qualitative data on the impact of context or moderator variables. Listed below are two examples of of such procedures.

Ecological Taxonomy of Intellectual Assessment

This informal procedure is the third in our bio-cultural assessment system and it was developed to gather descriptive information on children's skills and behaviors that are relevant to the context in which the child lives. The first component of the taxonomy uses a *behavioral observation procedure* to gather data on the child's behavior in multiple settings – the home and the school. Observing children's interactions with their family and friends allows the examiner to collect information about the family dynamics and the kinds of experiences in which they engage: their communication style, the kinds of activities in which they engage, how they approach tasks, and verbal expression with family members. The second component is the *Family/Community Support Questionnaire,* designed to ascertain what support systems the child has at home or in the community, what have been the child's educational experiences, the family's educational background, what language is spoken in the home, and involvement of the child and family in church/community organizations. The third component within the ecological taxonomy is the *Item Equivalencies Method*. It requires the examiner to review each item of the verbal subtests of the IQ test and match them to the child's culture when appropriate. In other words, the examiner should determine whether the concept being assessed has similar or equivalent meaning for children from culturally diverse backgrounds. And, finally, the fourth component within the ecological taxonomy is a *Teacher Questionnaire* that seeks information about the child, including his or her previous educational experiences, punctuality and absence histories, current academic performance in mathematics and reading, and levels of motivation and attention in class.

Assessment of Level of Acculturation

The impact of acculturation on performance on psychometric tests of intelligence has been well noted in the psychological assessment literature (Dana, 1993; Lewis, 1998; Sattler, 1992). It describes the extent to which individuals have retained their culture of origin or have adapted to the new culture (Casas & Casas, 1994; Phinney, 1996). In terms of assessment, the IQ test performance of an examinee from a culturally diverse background who lacks psychosocial adjustment to a new culture is not likely to be an accurate reflection of his or her true cognitive ability. To minimize the effects of acculturation on psychometric test performance, instruments have been developed to assess the examinee's level of acculturation. Typically, a checklist, rating scale, or questionnaire is used to seek information about an examinee's value orientations, language dominance and proficiency, prior knowledge, culture-specific attitudes, food practices, level of participation in ethnic organizations and traditional holiday celebrations. (See Cuellar, Arnold, and Maldonado, 1995; Dana, 1993; Landrine and Klonofff, 1994, for examples of acculturation measures.)

ASSESSMENT OF OTHER INTELLIGENCES

We support Gardner's thesis that individuals have more cognitive capacities than those measured on conventional IQ tests. We also share his contention that environmentally enriched contexts are likely to enable their nurturance or development. Toward that end, we developed the Other Intelligences Inventory as the fourth tier of the bio-cultural assessment system (Armour-Thomas & Gopaul-McNicol, 1998). It uses an interview format to gather information on four of Gardner's eight intelligences. Specifically, the examinee, the parents, and the teacher are asked questions to ascertain the examinee's musical, bodily-kinesthetic, inter- and intrapersonal intelligences.

CULTURE-REDUCING MEASURES

System of Multicultural Pluralistic Assessment (SOMPA)

This measure was developed by Mercer (1978) in response to a claim that too many children from culturally and linguistically diverse backgrounds were misclassified as mentally retarded and therefore erroneously placed in special education classes. It utilizes a system-oriented approach and incorporates three assessment models: medical, social system and pluralistic. The medical model assesses perceptual–neurological, nutritional and growth factors, physical dexterity, health history, and visual and auditory acuity. A medical examination and parental interview are used to gather information on these variables. The social system model assesses the degree to which a child is able to meet social expectations at school, at home, and in the community. The Wechsler Intelligence scales for children are used to assess the examinee's social role in school and the scores obtained are used to indicate the level of acculturation to the mainstream culture of the U.S. Two standardized parent interview procedures are used to answer questions about the social and cultural charcteristics of the family. The first one, the Adaptive Behavior Inventory for Children (ABIC), has six scales: Peer Relations, Nonacademic School

Roles, Family, Community, Earner/Consumer, and Self-Maintenance. The second interview procedure is the SocioCultural Scales, with four subscales: Urban Acculturation, Family Structure, Family Size, and Socioeconomic Status. And, finally, the pluralistic model uses information from the parent interviews to ascertain the Estimated Learning Potential (ELP) of the examinee and is based on comparison of the examinee with children from a similar sociocultural background.

Nonverbal IQ Tests

Nonverbal IQ measures, described in the literature as culture-free and culture-fair tests, were developed to reduce the language and culturally loaded content present in a test. In some sense, the term "culture-free" is a misnomer since any measure reflects, to some extent, the values, norms and expectations of a social group as well as an assumption that examinees have been socialized in the culture in which the test was developed. Among the more commonly used nonverbal tests are the Raven's (1938) Progressive Matrices, the Leiter (1948) International Performance Scale, and Cattell's (1973) Culture Fair Intelligence Test. Each is briefly described below.

The Raven's (1938) Progressive Matrices is a test of nonverbal reasoning. The examinee is presented with a set of figural matrices with one element missing and the examinee is required to choose the missing figure. It is often used for examinees with limited English proficiency or/and from ethnically and racially diverse backgrounds. Its non-speeded nature is considered culturally fair for some examinees whose cognitive functioning is negatively impacted by a speed factor.

Cattell's (1973) Culture Fair Intelligence Test is a multiple-choice paper-and-pencil measure that consists of four subtests: Series Completion, Classification, Matrices, and Conditions, which are highly speeded. It was designed to reduce the effects of educational and cultural experiences.

Leiter's (1948) International Performance Scale is a nonverbal measure and requires the examinee to choose pictures or blocks of symbols and to place them correctly. The test consists of 54 items grouped into seven categories: (a) spatial relations, (b) classification, (c) series completion and memorization, (d) picture completion, (e) design copying, (f) colors, shades, and pictures matching and (g) number estimation.

COMMENTARY

In response to the charge that conventional IQ measures do not accurately measure the intellectual functioning of children from culturally diverse backgrounds, this chapter has identified a number of culturally sensitive strategies and nonverbal measures—all intended to obtain a more precise estimate of an individual's intellectual performance. Although these procedures add valuable qualitative information about culture-specific issues in assesment, they are not without criticisms. The SOMPA, LPAD, and the Bio-Cultural Assessment System (B-CAS) require an enormous investment of time to administer and training of examiners. Also, questions have been raised about the validity and reliability of some of their subtests. For example, the absence of local norms for the Estimated Learning Potential of the SOMPA has been noted (Sattler, 1992). Validity studies need to be undertaken for the psychometric potential tier of the bio-cultural assessment system. Similar concerns have been raised about some of the nonverbal measures as well. For example, the administration of Cattell's (1973) Culture Fair Intelligence Test relies heavily on verbal instructions and thus may pose difficulties for children with limited English proficiency. Also, the highly speeded nature of some of its subtests may be problematic for some children whose cultures value time differently. Despite these shortcomings, these procedures, when used in conjunction with a conventional IQ test, do enable a more comprehensive understanding of intellectual functioning of children from culturally diverse backgrounds. Moreover, this multi-method approach yields more diagnostic information than a single IQ score and offers useful suggestions for educational interventions.

CONCLUSION

This chapter highlighted some of the more common charges of cultural bias in standardized tests of intelligence. We contend though that IQ tests can be used to guide educational decision-making and interventions if accompanied by other more culturally specific information. Toward this end, we identified some promising approaches, including our own bio-cultural assessment system. While none of these strategies can stand alone in providing reliable and valid information on an examinee's cognitive strengths and weaknesses, they do provide useful insights about the influence of culture on intellectual performance. Moreover, when used in conjunction with a conventional IQ measure, they yield information that can be used to inform prescriptive pedagogical interventions.

CHAPTER 6

Assessing the Linguistic Proficiency of Children from Culturally Diverse Backgrounds

INTRODUCTION

The increasing linguistic diversity among school-age children in the United States has made language proficiency a key construct in the assessment of children's academic and intellectual functioning. According to the United States Department of Education (1992) about 2.3 million children have been identified as "limited English proficiency." As a group, the number of children for whom standard U.S. English is not the language spoken in the home has grown in recent years. Olson (1993) reported that the number of K–12 children with limited English proficiency increased by 51.3 percent between 1985 and 1991. The presenting problem of linguistic diversity for equity in assessment is to differentiate whether the source of difficulty underlying observed behavior is due to disorders intrinsic to the individual or to cultural and linguistic differences. However, the disproportionate number of children from these backgrounds enrolled in special education classes (Lipsky and Gartner, 1996; Cummins, 1984) has led many to question the validity of results from standardized tests for this population of students

(Armour-Thomas, 1992; Gopaul-McNicol, 1992; Lidz, 1991; Figueroa, 1990; Oller, 1983).

Although Federal mandates (Equal Opportunities Act of 1974 and the Education for all Handicapped Children Act of 1975) and standards of professional organizations (e.g., American Psychological Association, 1985) set guidelines for the equitable treatment of language-minority students, these policies are difficult to implement. Nowhere is the difficulty more evident than in the measures used for assessing the communicative and linguistic functioning of this group of students. This chapter begins with a critical examination of extant standardized measures of language proficiency. During the course of this review, it will be shown how inattention to certain conceptual and methodological issues about language and culture has fueled the claim of bias in assessment for children socialized beyond the pale of the macroculture of the United States. Next, alternative or additional procedures will be explored with a view toward a more inclusive assessment system for language-minority school-age children.

STANDARDIZED TESTS OF ENGLISH LANGUAGE PROFICIENCY

A modular perspective of language proficiency underlies most tests of language proficiency (Hamayan and Damico, 1991). According to this view, language may be decomposed into discrete elements, each related to a particular domain of language structure and skills. Domains of structure include *speech* (articulation, voice, fluency) and *language* (receptive and expressive abilities). Moreover, this perspective assumes that these domains of speech and language and its subcomponents and skills are relatively autonomous and can be analyzed independent of the influence of cultural or extrinsic factors. Through the standardization process, decontextualized tasks in contrived settings are used to assess various components of language and communication. Data gathered from this discrete approach, as Carroll (1961) defined it, are then combined to yield an interpretation of the individual's overall communicative effectiveness. There are a number of standardized tests within a modular perspective that are currently in use that were designed for a monolingual English population. Some focus on the measurement of specific language structures (e.g., the Boehm Test of Basic Concepts (Boehm, 1971); the Peabody Picture Vocabulary test (Dunn and Dunn, 1982), the Carrow Elicited Language Inventory (Carrow, 1974)). Others have been designed to measure both specific abilities and other related language skills (e.g., the Illinois Test of Psycholinguistic Abilities and the Clinical Evaluation of Language Function (Semel & Wiig, 1987).

CONCERNS ABOUT ENGLISH TESTS OF LANGUAGE PROFICIENCY FOR ENGLISH LANGUAGE LEARNERS

Federal legislation and policies from professional associations require non-discriminatory assessment of children whose primary language is not English. This means that language proficiency tests currently intended for monolingual English populations are inappropriate for use with English-language learners (ELL). Over the years, conceptual and methodological concerns have been raised about the use of standardized measures of language proficiency for this group of students. Some of the more common criticisms are described next.

NARROW CONCEPTUALIZATION OF LANGUAGE

Some critics have argued that the modular perspective represents a narrow conceptualization of language and that it does not tell the full story of how normal language is used in everyday life. Instead, they claim that language is a dynamic semiotic system that functions in diverse communicative contexts and involves the total range of experiences within that context (Chomsky, 1956; Oller, 1989; Oller and Damico, 1991; Vygotsky, 1987). This view is based, in part, on empirical evidence that shows that normal language use involves meaning, and it is constrained by temporal factors (Oller, 1973; Savignon, 1983). In advancing a hierarchical model of language proficiency based on Oller's (1989) earlier work of pragmatic mapping, Oller and Damico (1991) proposed that the semiotic system comprises three interrelated subsystems (sensory–motor, kinesic and linguistic), each with its own associated grammatical structure that, in turn, corresponds to a particular genre of textual representations in experience. The acquisition of the conventional aspects of any given grammatical structure depends, in part, on the individual's ability to understand the text* in that particular subsystem at a sufficient level of detail. However, language proficiency is enabled by the interdependence of all three systems. These notions of language as an integrated system that functions holistically imply that to understand an individual's language proficiency requires an examination of the individual's exposure to different language structures that, in turn, may give rise to the acquisition of different types of skills. As Damico (1991) so aptly describes:

* Text in this context means different modes of representation (e.g., visual, auditory images, words, gestures).

> language and communication are revealed because some aspect of meaning,
> coded by grammatical structures for some purpose, is needed in a particular situa-
> tion (p. 178).

It follows from this synergistic perspective of language that tests designed to
assess language as numerous bits and pieces of decontextualized specific abilities lack construct validity since such measures ignore or undervalue manifestations of language developed through different experiences within different
cultural contexts. We elaborate upon these ideas further in a later section.

UNDERESTIMATION OF THE INTERDEPENDENCY OF LANGUAGE AND CULTURE

Investigators from diverse disciplines consider that language and culture,
though theoretically distinct, are so interrelated that it is difficult to differentiate the acquisition of language from the acquisition of culture. In explaining
how this interdependency unfolds, Och and Schieffelin (1984, p. 277) contend
that: (1) The process of acquiring language is deeply affected by the process of
becoming a competent member of society; and (2) the process of becoming a
competent member of society is realized, to a large extent, through language,
by acquiring knowledge of its functions, social distribution, and interpretations in and across socially defined situations, i.e., through exchanges of language in particular situations. Other studies of child language socialization
from cognitive anthropology and sociolinguistics point to both the importance
of language for acquiring and communicating the knowledge and skills of culture and also to how the very act of learning linguistic rules and routines
simultaneously involves the learning of culturally sanctioned ways of thinking
(Bruner, 1983; Heath, 1983; Quinn and Holland, 1987).

Harkness (1990) used the metaphor of "developmental niche" to provide a
theoretical framework for conceptualizing about the mechanisms by which the
child acquires and uses language in sociocultural settings. Harkness contends
that the developmental niche comprises three subsystems: (a) the physical and
social settings of the child's everyday life; (b) customs of child care and child-
rearing that are culturally sanctioned; and (c) the psychology of the caretaker. It
is hypothesized that these three components of development work together as a
system to regularize the child's environment, including language, and to mediate the child's experience within the larger culture. And it is in the process of
such mediated interaction that the child abstracts not only the rules of culture
but also the rules of language and its uses for representing experience to the self
and communicating about it to others. This conceptualization of the closely
related connection between acquisition of language and culture renders meaningless any discussion of language proficiency outside a culture's definition of its
own language tools and norms of discourse for organizing and communicating
knowledge to its members. Language measures developed in the U.S., with their

emphasis on the assessment of decontextualized language skills, are likely to favor children whose language socialization and acquisition were influenced by experiences within the mainstream culture. In this sense, while reliable and valid for children socialized according to the norms and values of the mainstream English-speaking culture of the U.S., these tests are invalid for children whose primary language socialization and acquisition occurred in other cultures.

IGNORING VARIATION IN LANGUAGE USE

Numerous factors can affect language variation such as socioeconomic level, ethnicity, recency of arrival in a new country, educational orientation, and regionality. In describing the tremendous variation in language use among Caribbean countries, Irish and Clay (1995) reported that Creole languages represented a cross-fertilization of African and European cultural influences to a large extent.Gopaul-McNicol, (1997) make a similar point about the African and U. S. cultural influences on the speech patterns of some children of African ancestry. As a result of these cultural influences, variation in a linguistic language system can occur both within the receptive and expressive domains and within subcomponents of each one (e.g. phonology, semantics, pragmatics, syntax, morphology). For some children the structural coding of meaning is most obvious at the phonological level. For example, Gopaul-McNicol (1997) reported that in Black dialects final consonants are often deleted or reduced so that the word "best" is pronounced "bes". Similarly, the differences between vowels "i" and "e" may not be maintained such that "tin" and "ten" are pronounced the same like "tin" in White dialects. Brereton (1995) identified variations among other domains of language structure:

> lack of verbal inflection, e.g. past tense is not marked by the use of ed.
>   The verb remains in its infinitive form;
> use of doz (does) before the verb to indicate a present habitual action;
> use of yustu (used to) before the verb to indicate a past habitual action;
> pluralization of differences: the plural is not indicated by the addition of
>   -s or -es. The plural may be indicated by the suffix dem (sometimes
>   spelled them) after the noun to be pluralized. (pp. 15–16)

It is easy to see how some examiners may regard these variations in language use as symptomatic of a problem more intrinsic to the individual. But, Irish and Clay (1995) cautioned that despite these surface differences Caribbean Creole speakers

> possess a rich storehouse of rich and complex language and cultural experiences
> that can be drawn on in the assessment process (p. 14)

Variation in language use also exists in the conventions and courtesies of conversation within and across various cultural groups. Tharp (1989) contrasted the discursive manner of speaking of the Navajo culture with the overlapping speech of the Hawaiian culture. Also Brice-Heath, (1989) described how the oral communicative practices of African American children from working class background were largely adaptive to community needs but were different from the expectations and practices of schools and the workplace. According to Brice-Heath, children learn oral skills for negotiating, interpreting and adapting to changing contexts, speakers and caregivers. And finally, Gauvain (1995) reviewed various research studies that showed how the ways of speaking are influenced by cultural conventions which are themselves used for organizing and communicating knowledge of a culture. Neither the norms nor the scoring of standardized tests of language reflects these variations in language use. More importantly, performance that deviates from standard English is interpreted negatively. Indeed, many researchers have expressed concern that negative attitudes toward English language learners may result in misidentification and placement in special education inappropriately (Irish and Clay, 1995).

MISDIAGNOSIS OF THE SOURCE OF THE LANGUAGE DIFFICULTY

Observed difficulty in language proficiency is frequently the reason for referral of the English language learners for assessment. The task of the examiner is to determine whether the difficulty is due to normal problems associated with second-language acquisition or to problems reflective of a language disorder or impairment. Hamayan & Damico (1991) identified at least two factors that may complicate the assessment process for this group of students in ways that could lead to a misdiagnosis of the source of the observed difficulty: similarities in problematic behaviors, complexity of second-language acquisition. Each will be elaborated upon briefly.

Similarities in problematic behaviors: The ELL population demonstrates behaviors similar to those observed in language-impaired monolingual English speakers (e.g. grammatical errors, mistakes in phonology and problems in comprehension).

Complexity of the process of second-language acquisition: They identified five features of second-language that may indicate inadequate language development in monolingual speakers but are normal manifestations of second-language acquisition:

interlanguage: an internal language system characterized by a combination of the students native language rules, English rules, or rules adapted from either or both languages;
code switching: a speech pattern that involves shifting between grammatical systems;

rule fossilization: maintenance of a less than perfect interlanguage system a condition related less to the learner's intrinsic learning capacity than to his/her motivations and experiences;

linguistic interference: misuse of vocabulary, errors in grammar, syntax, pronounciation of the native language which using the second language;

language loss: diminution of proficiency in a first language during second-language acquisition as a function of impoverished bilingual environmental factors.

Since these factors are common indicators of some aspect of impairment or poor language development among monolingual English speakers, but normal in second-language learners, a misdiagnosis can be made by an untrained examiner.

Inadequacy of Translations and Use of Interpreters

Direct translation of English tests of language proficiency into other languages is a common strategy used when assessing students whose primary language is not English. (See Damico, 1991 for a discussion of translation of tests of receptive and expressive language.) This is done to address concerns about linguistic and construct equivalence in test items for non English populations. But, ensuring equivalence is not an easy undertaking because of within-language variations in terms of dialectical and idiomatic expressions, and the difficulty of finding literal equivalents in the targeted languages. Moreover, the rules for ensuring that words have the same level of difficulty, same frequency of use, same meaning are difficult to maintain in translation. Others have noted similar concerns about translations (Dana, 1993; Lopez, Lamar and Scully-Demartini, 1997; Sattler, 1992).

Another common strategy involves the use of interpreter during the assessment process to minimize the potential linguistic and cultural bias of English tests of language proficiency. However, due to poor selection and training of interpreters difficulties may arise. For example, in translating items during the actual administration of the test, errors may occur in terms of omission, substitution or addition of words or phrases that may significantly change the content of the items (Lopez et. al 1997).

Toward A More Integrated Approach to Assessment of Language Proficiency

The different kinds of problems inherent in current standardized tests of language proficiency suggest the need for change. The synergistic perspective of language proficiency as a dynamic and integrated representational system that functions differently in different contexts provides conceptual direction for a more effective approach to assessment than what currently exists. The bio-cultural perspective of human development proposed earlier is in some ways compatible with the synergistic theory language proficiency and representational capacities as put forth by some researchers. For example, we share Oller and Damico's (1991) view that to some extent representational capacities are innate, and species-specific. We don't think though, that the empirical evidence is sufficiently compelling for their claim of an underlying general semiotic capacity that unites the three representational systems. Nor do we believe in the evolution of language development toward some endpoint that is universal across cultures. Rather, we concur with Harkness (1990) that:

> universal human capacities are differentially channeled to varying outcomes for representing experience to the self and communicating about it to others. (p. 728)

It seems to us that each representational capacity (sensory-motor, kinesic, and linguistic) is related to some degree to allow for the intertranslatability of experience from one modality to the next. However, associated with each bio-logically-derived representational capacity is a dynamic disposition and a synergy to develop to its fullest possible expression. Which representational capacity gets developed optimally, which ones atrophy, which ones develop simultaneously is a function of the nature and quality of stimuli within any given cultural niche at any developmental point in time as well as the sociopolitical forces operating within the larger culture. In other words, a culture's value system as well as the opportunities and constraints operating within these micro and macro cultures dictate what icon (sensory motor), index (kinesic) or symbol (linguistic) representational system/s is used to enable the development of language. To the extent that social, personal and material resources are available in a consistent manner in the language environment of the child, positive outcomes can be expected. Conversely, inadequate resources or adequate resources inconsistently deployed could adversely affect the course of language development.

It follows from these considerations about representational capacities and language development that it is necessary that assessment procedures examine multiple sources of evidence that characterize the kinds of experiences that may have produced the observed language behavior at a particular point in time. In addition, such assessment probes should also be accompanied by rich descriptions of the multiple contexts that define the sociocultural milieu in which the child grows and functions. The goal is to make a determination about relative strengths and weaknesses of the child in terms of language proficiencies from information gathered about his/her functioning through multiple modalities.

Methodologically, it is unlikely that any one measure could adequately assess language proficiency conceived this way since different contexts and experiences within them may call for the use of different grammmar structures and processes to accomplish particular goals at particular points in time. There are other complicating factors as well. A fundamental purpose of language assessment (e.g., to make comparisons about children linguistic proficiency) may necessitate a standardization of the assessment process so that quantitative information may be generated from which normative judgments about observed differences in language behavior may be made. To the extent though, that placement decisions are based on such comparative data, care must be taken to ensure that the equity principle is not violated. In other words, applying the equity principle in assessment requires that *all* children regardless of the backgrounds from which they come be given necessary and sufficient opportunities to demonstrate their competence. To the extent that assessment measures by design and administration favor a particular sociocultural experience over another, then the resulting data are likely to be valid for some but invalid for others. Such inequitable practices are likely to be reinforced or extended if decision makers use faulty data to make high-stakes decisions that could have far-reaching implications for the quality of some children's future life chances. To limit bias in standardized linguistic assessment would require an assessment system sufficiently inclusive to accommodate analysis of language behavior using both standardized and non-standardized measures. These measures should: appraise language proficiency under standardized conditions, ascertain language potentials that standardized measures may unwittingly mask, explore other manifestations of communicative competence and language proficiency in other contexts. In the section that follows we examine these concerns in more detail.

PSYCHOMETRIC LANGUAGE ASSESSMENT

When children for whom English is not the primary language or as Lacelle-Peterson and Rivera (1994) call them, " English Language Learners" (ELLs) are referred for evaluation the presenting problem is usually related to a communicative or language difficulty that the examinee is experiencing in the school context, more particularly, the classroom. First, the examiner administers a standardized language measure or battery to determine language dominance. Next, the examiner selects measures to assess various components and subcomponents of the student's dominant speech (articulation, voice and fluency); and expressive and receptive abilities (pragmatics, semantics, syntax, morphology and phonology). A standardized English language proficiency test *and* a translated version of the English test/or a proficiency test in the examinee's native language may be used for this purpose. Any of these measures will provide information on the examinee's developed ability to show his/her linguistic competence on de-contextualized tasks of speech and language in a contrived setting. Knowing the examinee's strengths and weaknesses in these areas is important for these are the kinds of basic linguistic competencies expected of children in formal school settings.

ASSESSMENT OF LANGUAGE POTENTIAL

During the course of the standardized administration, the examiner, on the basis of prior experiences with English Language Learners may make a decision to "step away" from standardized procedures to elicit language potentials not readily discernible within the standardized assessment context. At least three modifications may be made to accommodate the needs of English Language Learners. (a) *Suspending time.* Extra time may be allowed the examinee before responding to timed-questions. It is well documented that the concept of time does not mean the same thing for children socialized in cultures other than the mainstream English speaking culture of the United States. Some children may also need more time to translate an item from English into the examinee's own language and to translate the response back into English. (b) *Code switching.* This involves the shifting from one grammatical system to another when responding to test items. Researchers in the sociolinguistic tradition have noted that some bilingually proficient children code switch without violating the rules of both languages (e.g. Ramirez, 1985; and Irish and Clay, 1995). The examiner should make the clinical judgment whether to allow code switching for those examinees who may feel more comfortable or communicate more effectively using this feature of speech. (c) *Linguistic equivalence.* Words and phrases in English may convey different meanings in other non English speaking cultures. As such the examiner may need to use equivalent linguistic content when necessary in an effort to minimize the bias in test items. Other children because of their socialization experiences in the home or their peer group may experience difficulty in expressing vocabulary knowledge spontaneously. However, when asked to make a sentence using the word, such children are able to do so quite readily suggesting that the difficulty may be due to cultural factors rather than a problem more intrinsic to the children.

Ecological Approaches to Assessment

Through an analysis of the data gathered so far, the examiner would be able to generate a profile of observed strengths and weaknesses of the student in terms of performance of discrete skills associated with the domains of speech and language. But this information is insufficient for making interpretation regarding the source of the communication or language difficulty. Are low scores due to a cultural difference, a dialectical difference, learning English as a second language or something more intrinsic to the individual such as communicative/language impairment? Answers to these questions are likely to be answered through the assessment of speech and language in contexts where authentic conversations occur between and among individuals about meaningful tasks. Cultural niches where such person-task interactions relevant for the appraisal of effective communication include the home, the community and of course, the school. There are two levels of analysis for data gathered through ecological approaches. The first level of analysis seeks to determine the individual's proficiency in communication skills in what Damico (1991) calls oral monological use, oral dialogic language use and the use of contextually constrained communication. The second level of analysis seeks to distinguish problematic behaviors associated with language impairment from those that are related to normal difficulties in second-language acquisition. Procedures for each level of analysis would be considered in turn.

LEVEL 1 ANALYSIS

Procedures at this level are intended to assess communicative competence: in speech (articulation, voice and fluency) and language (receptive and expressive skills). Damico (1990) calls them "descriptive analysis procedures". Included among the more commonly uses approaches are the following: *screening approaches* (Chappell, 1980; Hamayan, Kwiat, & Perlman, 1986; Irish and Clay, 1995); *"story grammar" analyses* (e.g. Peterson and McCabe, 1983); *language sampling procedures* (Larson and McKinley, 1987; *rating scales or protocols* (Damico and Oller, 1985); behavioral observations (Calvert and Murray, 1985; Damico, 1985); *classroom discourse analyses* and *"cloze techniques"*(Simon, 1989; Laesch and van Kleeck, 1987). Damico (1991) describes three major manifestations of speech and language enabled through such ecologically-sensitive assessment:

> oral monologic communication: demonstration of static, dynamic relationships among objects and people as well as communication of abstract ideas;
>
> oral dialogic communication: demonstration of behaviors indicative of effective, fluent, and appropriate meaning transmission in conversational discourse;
>
> contextually-constrained communication: demonstration of behaviors indicative of appropriate oral communicative interactions within the academic setting.

Taken together these procedures will yield a rich source of data from which accurate judgments may be made with respect to speech and language communicative effectiveness. If a difficulty in one or more of these manifestations of performance is observed, then the examiner will need to engage to probe deeper for possible language impairment or other disabilities intrinsic to the individual.

LEVEL 2 ANALYSIS

Approaches at this level are intended to ascertain whether the difficulties observed in level 1 analysis are attributable to language learning disorders or to normal developmental problems associated with second-language acquisition. Damico (1990) referred to these approaches as "explanatory analysis procedures" and suggested that they involve two components: (a) procedures that gather data on the background of the student and the multiple contexts in which the student interacts (e.g., *interviews* with family and community members who are well acquainted with the student's current academic, social and family circumstances; *questionnaires* for evaluating the educational context of the student; *observational scales* and protocols that describe the functioning of family members in their home environment; and *ethnographic methods* to capture the student's functioning in multiple contexts); and (b) procedures that embody questions that help the clinician to localize the source of the problematic behaviors in communication. Damico (1991) gave some examples of these questions:

1. Are there any overt variables that immediately explain the communicative difficulties in English?
2. Does the student exhibit the same kinds of problematic behavior in the first language as in English?
3. Is there evidence that the problematic behaviors in English can be explained according to normal second-language acquisition or dialectical phenomena?
4. Is there any evidence that the problematic behaviors noted in English can be explained according to cross-cultural interference or related cultural phenomena?

CONCLUSION

The English language is the official medium of communication in the United States. Children from culturally and linguistically diverse backgrounds attending schools in the U.S. are at a decided disadvantage compared with their English-speaking peers. Difficulties in classroom discourse interactions and poor academic performance are the usual indicators of a potential problem in English language proficiency. However, despite their psychometric rigor for English-speaking children, standardized language tests are not sufficiently sensitive to locate the source of the difficulty in observed communicative performance of children from diverse cultural backgrounds. Variation in language use, complicating factors associated with second-language acquisition, and lack of native-language proficiency are but a few of the variables making interpretation of low language scores ambiguous. The increasing numbers of English language learners in schools entitled to equitable services, combined with the growing dissatisfaction with standardized tests for this population of students, are challenging policymakers to consider approaches beyond psychometric assessment. A number of contextually sensitive procedures have been proposed that hold promise for yielding more meaningful data on language proficiency for English-language learners than what obtains with current standardized language tests.

CHAPTER 7

Assessing the Academic Performance of Children from Culturally Diverse Backgrounds

A distinguishing feature of current discussion of educational reform is its dual focus on academic excellence and equity. Setting high standards for all students, irrespective of their cultural background and prior academic achievement, is seen as a key strategy toward these laudable ends at the national, state, and district policy levels in U.S. education. Targets have been established for what all students are expected to know and be able to do and curriculum frameworks in a variety of academic domains have been developed as well. To some extent, changing conceptions of student learning that focus more on higher-order thinking and problem-solving and less on decontextualized skills provide the theoretical rationale for the new ways of thinking of academic standards and curricula innovations. While these reform initiatives may represent a genuine commitment to the twin ideals of excellence and equity, insufficient understanding of the nature of the problem of underachievement of low-income children from culturally diverse backgrounds will make difficult the fulfillment of the promises of education reform.

Historically, standardized achievement tests have been used to gauge educational progress and achievement. A well-documented finding in comparative studies of academic achievement is that children from low-income, race/ethnic, and linguistic minority backgrounds do less well on these measures than their affluent, culturally dominant peers (Gardner, 1992; Garcia and Pearson, 1994). Some proponents of standardized achievement tests interpret these data as proof of individual and group differences in academic abilities and use such results to make decisions about tracking, grade promotion, and placement in special education programs. However, there may be explanations other than low ability for poor academic performance of this population of students. Also, because of the negative academic, social, and emotional consequences of the use of standardized test data for placement decisions of these children as a group, many critics continue to question the validity of such measures for low-income children, whose cultural socialization is significantly different from their middle-class peers, who have been socialized within the mainstream culture.

The purposes of this chapter are (1) to discuss the problems with current interpretation and use of results of standardized achievement tests when applied to children from culturally diverse backgrounds and (2) to identify some innovative procedures and consider their usefulness with this population of students, who traditionally have not been well served by our educational system.

INTERPRETATION OF ASSESSMENT RESULTS

Low scores on standardized achievement measures, such as reading and mathematics, are usually taken as indicators of low ability, leading to the kinds of placement and treatment described in the previous section. However, the attribution for low scores may reside more in experiences and contexts inimical to the development and expression of academic competence than in some underlying deficiency in academic ability. Consider some of these factors:

LESS THAN PROFICIENT ENGLISH LANGUAGE SKILLS

When English language learners are assigned to mainstream academic programs based on satisfactory performance on tests of English language proficiency, it is sometimes mistakenly assumed that they possess the minimum linguistic competence to deal with the academic content of classroom work. However, as Cummins has argued (1984), there seems to be a conceptual difference between basic interpersonal communicative skills (BICS) and cognitive academic language proficiency (CALP). Doing well in academically challenging courses in history or English literature requires a level of mastery of the English language skills of reading, writing, speaking, and listening that may be problematic for many English language learners. These learners may have the conceptual understanding of academic material in their native language but appear "not smart" when demonstration of such competencies is expected on standardized achievement tests in English.

LIMITED PROFICIENCY IN NATIVE AND SECOND LANGUAGE

Some children do poorly in school because they lack proficiency in both their native language and English. Skutnabb-Kangas and Toukomaa (1979) coined the term "semilingualism" to describe this deficiency in both languages. Some researchers (e.g., Cummins, 1984) caution that children who negotiate their academic environment with a very low level of proficiency in one or both languages will tend to experience academic difficulties. Understandably, without these foundational skills, children will predictably do poorly on any academic measure in English, even when the material is translated into the individual's native language. There are other factors that may exacerbate the situation for this group of children. Many of them have educational histories that show interrupted schooling and therefore may not have had the opportunity of developing the native language proficiency that comes with formal instruction. Others may come from homes with families who have recently arrived in the U.S. and who may not have the wherewithal to provide their children with the kinds of learning experiences conducive to dual language proficiency.

DIFFERENTIAL PRIOR EDUCATIONAL EXPERIENCES

A well-documented fact in cognitive psychology is the critical role of prior academic knowledge and skills in the acquisition of new knowledge and skills. Children with low scores on standardized achievement tests may not have had the perquisite knowledge and skills in the particular academic domains that current assessment presumes. We have already identified the absence of academically stimulating experiences and conditions for low-income, ethnic/race, and linguistic minority children placed in low-tracked and remedial classes as a result of low academic test scores. It should not be surprising that performance of these children on subsequent standardized achievement tests remains predictably low when comparisons are made with their high-track peers. Thus, it is through this cyclical process of placement–assessment–placement that standardized assessment serves to reinforce inequity in the educational opportunities that its initial results established in the first place! Other researchers have made similar claims about the unintended but negative consequences of standardized assessments in limiting some students' opportunities to learn (Darling-Hammond, 1991; Glaser, 1990).

INADEQUATE OPPORTUNITIES AND CONDITIONS TO LEARN

An enduring problem of underachievement of children of color from low-income backgrounds has been well chronicled in the educational and research literature. At-risk factors within the students themselves (Jensen, 1969; Herrnstein and Murray, 1994) and/or the debilitating circumstances of their lives (La Rosa and Maw, 1990; Walberg et al., 1988) have been common attributions offered for the problem. However, growing recognition among policymakers of inadequate schooling conditions and poor quality of services for this population of students have refocused attention on other sources for the problem of underachievement as manifested on standardized tests of academic achievement. Consider the data compiled by the Education Trust (1998) on teaching minority children from low-income backgrounds:

- they are often taught by the least prepared teachers;
- they are less likely to be enrolled in rigorous courses;
- they are too often treated differently in what they are expected to do and the kinds of assignments they are given, and;
- those who teach in high-poverty schools often lack the resources they need to teach well.

Similar findings regarding the differential quality of teaching for minority students attending high-poverty schools have been reported by others (e.g., The National Commission on Teaching and America's Future, 1996; Oakes, 1990; Gamoran et al., 1995). Is it any wonder that these students' performance on standardized tests is poor compared with their peers who have had better opportunities and conditions for learning?

OTHER PSYCHOCULTURAL FACTORS IN ACADEMIC UNDERACHIEVEMENT

Difficulties with language proficiency and inadequate prior knowledge are not the only reasons for low achievement. By now, it is well established that children from culturally diverse backgrounds experience school differently.

Earlier, some researchers used the concept of cultural deprivation to account for these differences, arguing that the experiences within the cultures of some ethnic minority children were deficient (Bereiter and Engelman, 1966; Deutsch, 1965). However, differential influences of socio-cultural forces on the lives of some children and their families, as well as differences between the culture of the home and the school, have replaced the deficit explanation of educational underachievement. We consider these issues in greater detail in the next section.

Hegemonic Values of the Macro Culture

Cultural reproduction theory, advanced by Bourdieu and Passeron (1977), remains one of the more persuasive arguments in accounting for the academic differences between children from low-income, race/ethnic, and linguistic backgrounds and their more affluent, English-speaking counterparts. According to this view, cultural elements mediate the relationship between capitalist structures operating in the larger society and the daily lives of people located in different class positions in the society. Through the process of socialization, children of the dominant class acquire different cultural knowledge, skills, linguistic competencies, and styles of interaction than do children from working-class backgrounds. But it is the cultural capital of children of the dominant class that is accepted by the dominant culture and which the educational system of the school requires of its students for academic success. Through its educational program, the school implicitly rewards the cultural capital of children from the dominant classes and systematically ignores or devalues that of working-class children.

Resistant Belief System of Microcultures

While not denying the role of capitalist structures and forces in the larger society and the collusion of the school system in maintaining the status quo, other researchers point to a resistant belief system of children of low-income, race/ethnic and linguistic backgrounds as an important variable in their academic underachievement. For example, Ogbu (1987) contends that African-Americans and Latinos from working-class backgrounds equate schooling with assimilation into the dominant culture, which they actively resist. These "caste-like minorities," as Ogbu calls them, exhibit patterns of behavior that are oppositional to the value system of the dominant culture and the school system. In other words, they refuse to adopt standard behaviors and attitudes that enhance school learning since they consider such practices as "acting white." Other researchers report the same phenomenon among Native American students (Kramer, 1991; Philips, 1983). In short, it is this resistant ideology and its associated oppositional behaviors that contribute to poor academic achievement of some low-income, race/ethnic, and linguistic minority children.

Cultural Incompatibility Between Home/Community and School Cultures

A classroom environment that expects rigid conformity to school norms reflective of a middle-class, Anglo cultural frame of reference, misunderstandings will arise between teacher and children whose cultural socialization differs significantly from their teachers. Such misunderstandings can contribute to academically non-productive classroom behavior that, in turn, may lead to academic underachievement. There is some research that indicates that in the natal Hawaiian culture, a common participation structure is for children to "co-narrate" a story with the principal speaker. In school, however, this overlapping communication style may be construed as "interrupting." When teachers were made aware of these cultural differences and adapted their reading programs to match the conversational style of the children, classroom reading improved (Au, 1980; Tharp, 1989). Sources of misunderstanding may also arise due to sociolinguistic differences between teacher and students. White and Tharp (1988) found that an Anglo teacher unintentionally interrupted Navajo children when they were speaking, mistaking a pause to mean that they were finished speaking. In another study, however, the researchers found increased participation among Pueblo Indian children when the teachers waited a little longer to respond to children's comments. (See Tharp's (1989) psychocultural variables and constants for a more comprehensive discussion of these differences.)

Difficulties in Acculturation

The term "acculturation" is sometimes used to describe a process of second-culture acquisition (LaFromboise, Coleman, and Gerton, 1993) or as the product of learning a culture that arises when members of two or more cultural groups come in contact with each other (Marin, 1991). Because the conditions under which cultural groups meet are negative (e.g., colonization, invasion, or conquest), the process may result in attitudinal and behavioral changes that are psychologically problematic. The level of identification with the value system of the culture of origin and the intensity of the emotional and affective feelings, may make adjustment to the host culture difficult. For immigrant children whose native language is not English, and who occupy a subordinate class position in the host culture, the adjustment is particularly difficult. Indeed, as Lynch (1992) observed, some children experience culture shock in the host culture when they unsuccessfully attempt to use communicative patterns and problem-solving strategies common in their natal culture. These problems manifest themselves in a school setting where, as a result of miscommunication and misinterpretations, school professionals mislabel some children from culturally diverse backgrounds as uncooperative, uncommunicative, or unmotivated (Lopez and Gopaul-McNicol, 1997).

USE OF STANDARDIZED TEST RESULTS

Standardized test data are often used as a basis to track and retain students and to place them in special education programs. These policies have had negative consequences for children, particularly those from culturally and linguistically diverse backgrounds. Inattention to these issues diminishes the likelihood that the lofty goal of equity and excellence for all will be attained. We elaborate on these concerns next.

TRACKING

Over the last twenty years, a consistent finding of many studies is that a disproportionate numbers of low-income, race/ethnic and linguistic minority students have been placed in low-tracked classes where opportunities for optimal learning are seriously diminished, leading to serious questions of the legitimacy of this practice. Consider some of the evidence:

Teachers of low-track classes fragment topics into isolated bits of information in such a way that lessons lack overall coherence (Oakes, 1985).

Assignments require rote memorization and little of such critical thinking skills as abstract reasoning and problem solving (Oakes, 1985).

The classroom environment is less conducive to learning than it is in high-track classes (Allington, 1980).

The emphasis is more on memorizing instead of problem solving and understanding (Good and Brophy, 1994).

Teachers spend less time on instruction and more on behavior management (Oakes, 1985).

Curriculums focus on low-level skills and less rigorous topics (Nystrand and Gamoran, 1988).

Other analyses of the tracking system have revealed that placements often parallel race and class differences. For example, the College Board (1985) found that Black students are more likely than White students to be enrolled in lower-track vocational and general programs. Low-income and minority students are more likely to be judged as having "low ability" and to be placed in remedial, special education, or low-track classes (Persell, 1977; Slavin, 1987). Oakes' (1990) analysis of science and mathematics education revealed a similarly disturbing pattern. She found that at all levels of schooling—elementary, junior, and senior high schools—minority children from low-income backgrounds were disproportionately placed in low-track classes.

GRADE RETENTION

Some states use standardized test results to retain children who have not mastered coursework for their current grade placement. More than ten years ago, Shepard and Smith (1986) found that academic achievement did not improve substantially following retention. Furthermore, repeating a grade had a negative impact on children's self-esteem and social adjustment. More recently, (Darling-Hammond, 1994) found similar evidence of negative impact of grade retention and cautioned that its adverse academic and social consequences increased the likelihood of children dropping out of school.

SPECIAL EDUCATION

The overrepresentation of low-income children from culturally diverse backgrounds in special education classes remains one of the serious criticisms of the use of standardized tests for making placement decisions. Consistent with earlier findings, an analysis of Department of Education data by U.S. News & World Report ("Separate and Unequal," 1993) found that Blacks are twice as likely as Whites to be in special education programs. A similar pattern of over-representation is found at the local school district as well for Black and Latino students as well (Lipsky & Gartner, 1996). The finding of very high correspondence between teacher referrals and final special education placement (Shepard and Smith, 1986) and the inappropriateness of such referrals for ethnic-language minority students (Irish and Clay, 1995) lead some educators to believe schools are unable to educate well this population of students. According to Richardson, (1994)

> Studies show teachers refer kids who bother them, and we've been able to demonstrate that specifically African-American males demonstrate behavior that bothers teachers (p. B7).

TOWARD A MORE NON-DISCRIMINATORY APPROACH TO ACADEMIC ASSESSMENT

Low income children from culturally diverse backgrounds are doubly disadvantaged by the interpretation and use of standardized achievement test results.

The knee-jerk interpretation of low ability for poor academic achievement as measured by standardized tests betrays an incomplete understanding or an ignoring of the socio/cultural forces operating both in the larger society as well as in the home and the school that negatively impacts on the learning and performance of the majority of these children. Similarly, the absence of academic, social or emotional treatment benefits from tracking, grade retention and special education placement contributes to a continuing skepticism of the validity of standardized test data for this population of students. But these criticisms are not new. For example Messick (1989) has cautioned the standardized testing community that test validity cannot be understood apart from societal values and therefore the validation of test interpretation and use, in part, rests upon the evaluation of intended and unintended consequences of any testing. Indeed, it is because of this concern about the negative consequences of test results that there is now an expectation of assessment developers to show the *consequential validity* of their measures (Glaser, 1990; Shepard, 1993).

Because of the vulnerability of low-income children from culturally diverse backgrounds to misinterpretation and misuse of results of standardized achievement tests, we think that different purposes should be served by assessment. Rather than define limitations in ability, which are, in turn, used to justify inequitable educational opportunities, assessment should probe for manifest strengths and emerging potentials of these children. On the basis of such diagnostic information, intervention strategies should be explored for reinforcing observed strengths and for bringing nascent competencies into full bloom.

We make a similar argument for the development of academic ability as we did for language and intellectual ability. That is, children are born into this world with biologically constrained potentials that get differentially channeled as a result of exposure to experiences within cultural niches as well to other sociocultural forces operating in the larger society. How these potentials are developed, and the pathways along which they unfold, depend on particular aspects within these contextualized experiences and the individual's responsiveness to them. Applying this conceptualization to academic development requires a consideration of the person–task interactions occurring within cultural contexts, such as the school, peer group, the home, or any other context that could influence the academic functioning of the child. It also requires an examination of the opportunities and constraints operating within both the local cultural context and the larger society that could positively or negatively impact on the acquisition of academic knowledge, skills and attitudes. To the extent, then, that experiences within and across these multiple contexts are conducive to academic achievement, positive outcomes can be expected. Conversely, experiences not conducive to academic development will predictably lead to academic underachievement.

In drawing implications for equitable assessment of children's academic functioning, particularly those of low-income, ethnic, and linguistic minority backgrounds, it is crucial to examine multiple sources of evidence. Since children function in multiple cultural contexts simultaneously, sampling behaviors within them may shed light on the nature and quality of experiences that may have influenced the behavior observed at a particular point in time.

Methodologically, as with intellectual and language functioning, no one measure will suffice since person-tasks interactions may produce different kinds of academic knowledge and skills represented in different ways. There is a place for standardized achievement tests within any assessment system since such measures can provide useful *descriptive* information about the child's manifest cognitive functioning within a particular context, under particular conditions. Given what we know, though, about the unequal opportunities for quality teaching-learning experiences in most school systems in the U.S., comparative judgments or interpretations of performance in terms of high or low ability should be avoided. Other measures would be needed to appraise the academic potentials that standardized procedures mask but which would be important to elicit. And finally, assessment tools would need to ascertain academic performance derived from more authentic and meaningful academic experiences. In the next section we explore these issues further.

PREASSESSMENT ACTIVITIES

Before administering a standardized test of academic achievement, the examiner should gather information about the examinee's prior and current educational experiences, language proficiency in both native and English languages. A questionnaire and or/interview protocol may be used to gather information from family members about the educational background and linguistic competence. In addition, the examiner should conduct an observation of the examinee in the classroom to obtain information on variables that may help interpret results from the standardized academic achievement measure. Indeed, questions like the ones used for intellectual assessment may be used here as well.

Psychometric Academic Assessment

To establish the examinee's current level of general academic achievement a standardized test of achievement may be used. Such a test seeks to ascertain manifest strengths and weaknesses in specific content areas (e.g. science, mathematics, reading, social studies, language arts). Individually- administered norm-referenced tests include the Wide Range Achievement Test, the Peabody Individual Achievement Test, the Part 11 of the Woodcock- Johnson

Psychoeducational Battery and the Wechsler Individual Achievement Test. Standardized reading and math tests in non-English Languages may be used for English Language learners or children with limited English proficiency. Information obtained from any of these measures is useful for it offers general guidance with respect to instructional intervention.

Assessment of Academic Potential

The psychometric potential assessment is designed to yield supplementary information about academic functioning that goes beyond what is provided by the static measure of standardized academic achievement. During the course of the standardized administration of an individual achievement test (e.g. the Wechsler Achievement Test), the examiner, on the basis of clinical observation of the examinee's responses to questions may decide to "step away" from standardized procedures to elicit information about a student's academic potential. The examiner may decide to "test to the limits" by giving the child more time to complete a task. If, after utilizing the *Suspending Time* procedure, the examinee gets the item right, then the examiner would have ruled out conceptual difficulty as the reason for not completing the task within the standardized time limitation. Also, the examiner may decide to use the *Paper and Pencil for Arithmetic* procedure to ascertain whether the examinee has the conceptual mathematical knowledge and skill but could not manipulate the mathematics symbols without an external prop. For items that are unfamiliar to to the examinee, the examiner may use a test-teach-retest method to ascertain learning potential. And finally, the examiner may decide to use an alternative procedure- *Contextualization for Vocabulary* to assess the examinee's vocabulary if the examinee fails to respond when asked to give the meaning of decontextualized words.

ALTERNATIVE ASSESSMENTS

One response to criticisms of standardized tests of academic achievement is alternative assessments. These types of assessments use direct judgment and appraisal of student behavior. They are sometimes called "classroom-based assessments since they are used to judge student performance on classroom tasks that are themselves tied to curriculum standards. Such procedures enable teachers to gather information about what students' actually know and can do, the process of their thinking as well as the product of their thoughts. Furthermore, they offer students the opportunities to bring to the classroom knowledge and skills acquired in their out-of-school experiences and to apply their classroom knowledge and skills to real-world experiences (Armour-

Thomas, 1992; Baker, 1991; Resnick and Resnick, 1992; Wiggins, 1989). Students respond to tasks by generating solutions, communicating their problem solving strategies, creating products, giving oral reports, conducting an experiment, mounting an exhibition, etc. When appraisals are derived from observation of students actual performance or samples of their work, alternative assessments are called "performance assessments" (Garcia and Pearson, 1994). Proponents of these measures for students from culturally and linguistically diverse populations suggest that they are accommodating of diversity of learning styles (Gordon, 1999); cultural preferences for different ways of participating in classroom activities (Au, 1993; Delgado-Gaitan, 1987) that are not compatible with a standardized testing paradigm (Darling-Hammond and Goodwin, 1993). And there are some studies that show a narrowing of the race/ethnic gap in academic achievement (e.g., Newmann, Marks, and Gamoran, 1995; Newmann and Wehlagen, 1995; Supovitz and Brennan, 1997). The next section discusses two types of alternative assessments that are prevalent in the educational literature: curriculum-based assessments and portfolios.

CURRICULUM-EMBEDDED ASSESSMENT

As the name implies, curriculum-embedded assessment describes the assessment of instructional needs by measuring students' performance on the very tasks used for instruction (Gickling and Havertape, 1981). Four assumptions are central to this form of assessment: (1) assessment procedures are designed so that they mirror the nature of the current instruction; (2) assessment tasks are drawn from the instructional materials; (3) results from assessment tasks assist the teacher in remediating students' difficulties on materials previously covered; and finally (4) data from assessment tasks help the teacher to design more effective instructional strategies for subsequent coverage of instructional content. The process may be described as: assess, instruct, assess, instruct.... This iterative dynamic feedback function allows for on-line instruction and sensitivity to changes in student learning and performance. Arts PROPEL (Gardner, 1989) and Project Spectrum (Krechevsky and Gardner, 1990) are examples of curriculum-embedded assessment.

PORTFOLIO ASSESSMENT

A portfolio is an alternative assessment device for housing samples of student work collected over time from classroom assignments. As a self-evaluative tool for students, it allows them an opportunity not only to demonstrate what they know and can do but also to reveal their misconceptions or flaws in their thinking about academic tasks. In addition, it allows them an opportunity to show their improvements over time. As a monitoring device for the teacher, it provides direct evidence for their judgments of student work and a tangible basis for guiding instruction. Increasingly, states and districts are using portfolios as one component in their assessment system. For example, since 1990, the Rochester City School district (RCSD) has been using portfolios in mathematics and language arts in the primary grades.

COMMENTARY

Although alternative assessments have great appeal to educators for their promise in addressing the equity-related shortcomings of standardized tests, concerns remain. Difficulties of obtaining inter-rater reliabilities on classroom assessments and the prohibitive costs of developing, scoring and translating them for English-language learners are some of the unresolved challenges of alternative assessments. We contend, though, that these measures, when used in conjunction with standardized tests, provide a rich source of diagnostic information from which more meaningful interventions may be mounted.

CONCLUSION

Traditionally, standardized achievement tests have been used to make decisions on tracking, grade retention and placement in special education programs. Proponents justify their use on the grounds that such measures provide objective information about real individual and group differences in academic abilities. Critics, however, question the scientific legitimacy of this claim since judgments of low achievement test scores often parallel race, class, and language differences (Oakes, 1985; Cummins, 1984; Samuda, 1975). Moreover, the fact that a disproportionate number of children with these demographic characteristics are placed in low-track classes and show higher dropout and grade retention rates than their more affluent, white, English-speaking peers has strengthened the distrust of standardized tests for this population of students. Indeed, many researchers believe that the use of standardized tests may have the unintended consequences of limiting access to further learning opportunities for some children. In this chapter, we have also argued against the use and interpretations of standardized tests for children of low-income, race/ethnic, and language minority backgrounds and proposed a reconsideration of the purposes of assessment—a reconsideration that places a greater emphasis on the identification of learner strengths and emerging academic potentials. Toward that end, we proposed a bio-cultural perspective of academic achievement that includes the assessment of academic potential and alternative assessments.

CHAPTER 8

Assessing the Visual-Motor and Neuropsychological Functioning of Culturally Diverse Children

VISUAL-MOTOR ASSESSMENT

Two assumptions have guided the inclusion of visual-motor assessment with elementary school children: One posits that visual-motor skills are prerequisites for successful school performance and the other claims that learning disabilities are manifestations of visual-motor deficits (Cummings and Laquerre, 1990). Frostig and Maslow (1973) have managed to advance the notion that learning disability has its roots in perceptual pathology, and they have also proposed methods of remediating visual-motor deficits in children. Given the current emphasis on the prevalence of visual-motor deficits in learning disabled youngsters, it is critical that assessment be as accurate as possible, especially with culturally diverse children, who were rarely represented on most currently used standardized tests.

To a large extent, an examiner's philosophy on assessment determines the process by which they gather data (Cummings and Laquerre, 1990). The nomothetic approach to assessment relies on objective standardized tests and assumes that all individuals have had the same social and educational experiences.

The greatest criticism of the nomothetic approach is that "the scores overpower the clinician's report of the motivational and background factors, yielding a deviance score or an index of difference" (Cummings and Laquerre, 1990, p. 593). In contrast to this nomothetic orientation is the hypothesis testing approach (Kaufman, 1979) or the bio-cultural approach (Armour-Thomas and Gopaul-McNicol, 1997, 1998). These approaches propose that the examiner develop hypotheses about the child from multiple sources, namely, clinical observations of the child in various settings—the home, school, community, church, etc. Interviews with significant others, such as the teacher or parents, are also critical if utilizing this approach. Potential assessment, whereby the child's strengths are highlighted instead of the dangerous practice of searching for pathology, is encouraged. The authors all recommend a more eclectic, comprehensive, cultural approach to assessment.

This chapter addresses three areas; the first section examines the common assumptions underlying the existing practice of the most commonly used visual-motor assessment measure. The second section explores alternatives to these traditional approaches as they apply to culturally diverse children, and the third section offers some discussion on the limitations of these proposed alternative approaches.

TRADITIONAL ASSESSMENT OF VISUAL-MOTOR SKILLS—QUANTITATIVE APPROACH

The Bender Gestalt Motor Test has been recognized as one of the most useful tools in the assessment of neurological functioning (Ghassemzadeh, 1988). It is an instrument which measures perceptual motor development, visual-motor integration and motor coordination (Sattler, 1992; Taylor, 1984). Since its introduction, many scoring systems have been devised for use with the Bender Gestalt (Hutt, 1977). Of these scoring systems, the most widely used is that developed by Koppitz (1981), which has been used primarily as a screening instrument for neurological problems (Eno and Deitchmann, 1980) and the identification of perceptual motor deficits.

Ethnicity has been found to relate to the visual-motor performance of children (Connelly, 1983; Koppitz, 1975; Taylor and Partenio, 1984). Studies have shown that Black and Hispanic children perform lower than White children at almost every age level (Sattler and Gwynne, 1982). Unfortunately, the studies do not seem to offer any clues to account for these ethnic differences.

Robin and Shea (1983) found that the performance of children from varying cultural backgrounds on the Bender Gestalt Visual Motor Test may be related to differences in the experiences that the children had prior to the testing. The author did not agree with previous investigators who felt that the delayed performance of culturally diverse children on these perceptual motor tests is a result of delays in their cognitive development. Rather, the author concluded that the delays can be attributed to the familiarity or lack thereof with these types of tasks. Gilmore, Chandy and Anderson (1975) compared Mexican-American students with that of Caucasians on the Bender-Gestalt. Beginning at age 7, a noticeable trend for the Mexican-American subjects was observed by the researchers. More errors were made by this group than by their Caucasian counterparts. The authors attributed these differences to the way the groups responded to the demands for accuracy, order and conformity. The authors believed that Caucasian children learn and are rewarded for responding to these demands more than non-Caucasian students are. Snyder, Holowenzak, and Hoffman (1971) conducted a study of children from diverse cultural backgrounds and their performance on the Bender-Gestalt. The purpose of this study was to compare the relative frequencies of certain errors made on the Bender designs. The results indicated that six types of perceptual-motor reproduction errors were made by these first- and third-graders. Distortion, rotation and integration errors were made most frequently by third-graders. For first-graders, distortions of angles were the most frequent errors recorded.

Gopaul-McNicol (1993) administered the Bender Gestalt test of visual-motor integration to West Indian and West Indian-American children. It was found that most children made errors of rotation more than any other error. In testing the limits after the initial administration, these children were able to recognize that their designs were different from those of the original. Since on the Bender, rotations are scored as errors, leading to the labeling of some of these children as neurologically impaired or as having visual-motor deficits, it is imperative to consider a differential diagnosis since the clinical indicators purported by errors of rotation and distortion may not be applicable for West Indian subjects. The fact that the children were able to draw them correctly once taught to do so suggests that they visually perceive the designs differently due to a culturally different interpretation in visual perception rather than visual-motor deficits, as many psychologists erroneously conclude. It is obvious that the present findings lend support to the fact that Bender performance can be related to cultural influences and should be interpreted with caution for immigrant children. It may be necessary for school psychologists, when testing some immigrant children via the Bender test, to point out to the student after the initial administration of all nine Bender designs any rotation errors noted. Allotting extra time for re-drawing the designs is also suggested. This will aid in determining if errors are truly a clinical sign or a culturally different interpretation in visual perception.

Gopaul-McNicol (1993) also found that many of these West Indian children took approximately 15 minutes to complete all of the designs. Even when they were told to work quickly, they continued to work at a slow pace. Of course, this may be in keeping with the cultural customs of these children. The social awareness that "anytime is West Indian time" seemed to fit the unhurried attitude they took when told they were being timed. Therefore, psychologists may need to encourage West Indian students to work at a more rapid pace and refrain from making erroneous assumptions about students' motivational attitude.

Although several objective scoring systems have been developed for use with the Bender Gestalt Motor Test, each has been criticized as being inadequate in some form or another (Parsons and Lawner Weinberg, 1993). Neale and McKay (1985) claim that the Koppitz system is not as objective as is desired. They found that with the increase in number of raters for a set of protocols, the inter-rater reliability on an item-by-item basis decreased. In other words, raters had difficulty following the standard procedures set forth by the system, which resulted in disagreement pertaining to individual items. Brannigan and Brunner (1989) suggested that all elements of clinical judgment be incorporated into an objective scoring system—responding to both essentials of the Gestalt and the amount of differentiation of designs (Schacter, Brannigan, and Tooke, 1991).

CULTUROLOGICAL ASSESSMENT OF VISUAL-MOTOR SKILLS—QUALITATIVE APPROACH

Dean (1986) stated that the future of visual-motor assessment will rely less on objective data (an extension of the psychometric workup) and more on the need to understand the client's functional deficits—a more holistic, comprehensive, qualitative approach. In our experiences, more experienced clinicians tend to step away from the quantitative approach to assessing visual-motor skills to the more behavioral approach, that is, observing the client's behavior while the client is copying the designs (Cummings and Laquerre, 1990). Like these clinicians, we believe that it is the observation of the act that gives greater insight into the child's difficulties.

Sugar (1992) developed a new, as yet unpublished scoring system which incorporates both qualitative and quantitative components, focusing on remediating the aforementioned difficulties, and which, purportedly, can be used easily by non-trained educators and clinicians. The Sugar Scoring System utilizes six of the original nine Bender Gestalt designs (modified version) which are developmentally appropriate for five- to six-year-olds (Figs. A, 1, 2, 4, 6, and 8). As in the Koppitz System, scores on the quantitative component are based on integration, perseveration, rotation, distortion of shape, distortion of size and linearity. Scores on the qualitative components are based on the Gestalt of the six designs and on the strategies and mode of execution used, taking into account the number of times a child makes a qualitative error. A point system ranging from 0 to 1 point is given per design reproduction, with 0 points depicting failure and 1 point representing acceptable performance. A maximum total of six points can be obtained for the quantitative category. As previously discussed, the qualitative segment reflects overall Gestalt, strategy, and execution. A point system ranging from 0 to 2 points is allotted per criterion, with 0 points representing minimal quality and 2 points depicting maximum quality. After weighting the quantitative and qualitative scores, a single score, which is an average of the two components, is tabulated, with a mean of 100 and a standard deviation of 15. Parsons and Weinberg (1993) found that this new system has been shown to be psychometrically sound in validity and reliability. Because the Sugar scoring system is more sensitive to a clinical perspective than the Koppitz, Brannigan and Brunner (1992) and Parsons and Weinberg (1993) have recommended it as a better and reasonable alternative to the existing scoring methods of the Bender Gestalt for culturally different children. Besides, it seems to have more applicability in clinical, educational and research settings than the other scoring systems.

Gopaul-McNicol, Scully-Demartini, and Diaz (in progress) examined the visual-motor performance of 70 Hispanic children, ages 5:0 to 6:11 years, who were originally from Puerto Rico, the Dominican Republic, Ecuador, Colombia, or El Salvador. By utilizing the Bender Gestalt Visual Motor Test, two scoring systems—the Koppitz (1945) and Sugar (1992)—were examined to determine the best measure of visual-motor functioning. Although this study is currently under investigation, the current findings reveal that the Sugar scoring system yields a higher score than the Koppitz scoring system. It is possible that the combined quantitative and qualitative scoring system allows the child the opportunity to interject his/her cultural experiences into the testing situation. Thus, in assessing a child's perceptual motor functioning, a scoring system that takes into consideration the impact of culture via a qualitative approach ought to be a focus. As in intellectual assessment, a uni-modal approach (quantitative only) is not advised. Rather, a multimodal approach (quantitative and qualitative) with cultural considerations is recommended for greater accuracy in assessment and diagnosis.

DIFFERENTIAL DIAGNOSIS—ROTATIONS: A SIGN OF VISUAL-MOTOR DELAYS OR CULTURAL INTERPRETATION?

Gopaul-McNicol and Beckles (1992) found that children from the English-speaking Caribbean tended to rotate their designs the first time they were asked to draw them. After assessing 110 children from four English-speaking

Caribbean islands, the authors found that irrespective of age, gender, socioe-conomic status, and educational level, the children tended to rotate the designs. It was as if they were executing the designs to fit their own realm of cultural experiences. By observing the children, the authors also noted that they were able to self-correct with the minimum of intervention. For instance, by asking the children the following question: Is your design like mine?

If the child says no, simply ask the child to draw it like the examiner's; the authors found that many children drew the designs correctly with no further prompting. If it was a true clinical neurological impairment, the children would not have been able to correct their "errors" so easily. Clearly, the children tend to perceive the designs differently due to a culturally different inter-pretation in their visual perception than due to visual-motor deficits.

LIMITATIONS OF THE PROPOSED ALTERNATIVE CULTUROLOGICAL APPROACHES

Although it is our contention that, like all areas of assessment described thus far in this book, visual-motor assessment should be conducted in a contextu-al, behavioral, multimodal, process-oriented manner, which will afford the examiner the opportunity to observe the child's performance beyond a quanti-tative, product-like fashion, there are some limitations even with this approach that ought to be considered.

First, critics of this bio-cultural model have spoken against the extended length of time required to complete the entire four tiers in any given assess-ment. Is twice the time of the typical traditional psychometric test a realistic expectation for an examinee, especially a young child?

Not included in this chapter is how an examiner chooses a particular struc-tured visual-motor measure, considering there are so many theoretically, psy-chometrically, culturally, and clinically overlapping questions that must be addressed.

Along this vein, does translating a test to a non-English-speaking child result in uninterpretable results or gross misinterpretation (Brislin, 1986)? The emphasis throughout this book is the inappropriateness of assessment meas-ures that were developed on one population and used on another.

From a theoretical point, the bio-cultural model should be expanded to ask what is the domain being assessed; in other words, is there a normal range of functioning or is the assessment of abnormalcy more important? Therefore, the examiner should further examine whether the Bender test, in this case, closely matches the examiner's definition of the constructs of his/her own interests.

From a psychometric standpoint, the obvious question that should be examined is, is the psychometric potential assessment tool appropriate in and of itself? Is there adequate internal consistency reliability, such as test–retest reliability? Is there an adequate key for scoring? Can this assessment tool predict external criteria appropriately and do they demonstrate convergent and discriminant validity with similar subtests from other type assessment measures (Holden, 2000)?

In like manner, while it is quite appropriate to use this psychometric potential tool with the cultural groups on which the data were gathered, is it relevant to any culturally and linguistically diverse groups of children? In other words, can one generalize with this tool from its culture of origin to any culture from which the examinee came? Therefore, could this bio-cultural model withstand the very criticisms (inappropriately imposed etic approach), as opposed to a more emic type test that was espoused so vociferously with this model?

Finally, another concern by critics of this model is the relative normative data or lack thereof of the psychometric potential assessment. While this is a common criticism, the authors are cognizant that informal qualitative measures, such as the bio-cultural approach, can not have the same psychological rigors as standardized tests because of the emphasis on clinical observations and assessment in the child's natural environment.

IMPLICATIONS FOR TRAINING PSYCHOEDUCATIONAL EVALUATORS IN ADMINISTERING VISUAL-MOTOR TESTS

In general, training of psychologists and other educational evaluators should begin in their graduate training programs. Exposing students to the issues raised in this chapter and the alternative approaches to using traditional visual-motor measures should be done simultaneously with students being exposed to the psychometric type visual-motor tests.

A more detailed examination of critical training issues for school personnel in assessing the visual-motor functioning of minority populations is discussed in Chapter 12.

NEUROPSYCHOLOGICAL ASSESSMENT AND CULTURALLY DIVERSE CHILDREN

The assessment of a brain-damaged child is a complex and exacting task requiring extensive specialized knowledge. The goal of neuropsychological examinations is to assess brain-damaged children more accurately, especially in the area of higher-level cognitive dysfunction. With the continued increase of school-aged children being diagnosed with learning disability, it is necessary for school personnel to include in their evaluations possible underlying causes of neuropsychological impairments (Schacter Brannigan and Tooke, 1991). What makes this task particularly difficult is the cross-cultural manifestation of learning disability (Armour-Thomas and Gopaul-McNicol, 1997). Increased diagnostic precision in medicine and psychology should take into consideration the results of neuropsychological tests, so that less emphasis would be placed on identifying the etiology and more emphasis placed on the behavioral consequences of neurologically related disorders and the intervention techniques needed for remediation (Sattler, 1988). Neuropsychological evaluations may also assist in evaluating children with reading and other academic problems and neuropsychological tests provide behavioral information about the child's adaptive functioning, as well as the effects of varying therapeutic programs on cerebral functions. Thus neuropsychological tests help the examiner to draw inferences about the strengths and weaknesses of the child. Some questions the examiner may seek to answer from a neuropsychological examination might be the following:

1. Does the child have difficulty paying attention and following in the classroom?
2. Is this child a good candidate for a visual memory training group?
3. What is the best educational program for this child?

To answer these questions, we have to first refocus our discussion on the concept of attention, which is used widely by educators. Teachers demand attention from their students and psychologists/psychiatrists diagnose children as suffering from attention deficit disorder (ADD). Attention includes information that is neuropsychological in nature. Attention is a common prerequisite for learning and memory (Das, Naglieri, and Kirby, 1994).

Attention can be assessed by appropriate tasks which have been useful in distinguishing among children with special needs. For instance, The Posner Physical and Name Match Test, designed to match pairs of letters that are visually identical or items identical in name, has been used in constructing two sets of tasks, Picture Matching and Letter Matching. The cultural biases in these tests are evident by the types of pictures used, which often are unfamiliar to culturally diverse children. The bio-cultural assessment system allows for a more dynamic approach to assessment, so that item equivalencies can be explored by using more familiar pictures, as is recommended in the third tier (ecological assessment) of the bio-cultural assessment system. Again, in keeping with the second tier of the bio-cultural assessment system, time could be suspended instead of the timed format in the standard instruction.

THE USE OF THE BIO-CULTURAL MODEL IN NEUROPSYCHOLOGICAL TESTING

HALSTEAD REITAN NEUROPSYCHOLOGICAL TESTS BATTERY FOR CHILDREN

Halstead Reitan Neuropsychological Tests Battery for Children contains cognitive and perceptual motor tests. Some of these tests in their standard form are the Matching Picture Tests described above, Target Tests which require the child to reproduce a visually presented pattern after a three-second delay, and the Tactile Form Recognition which requires the child to identify various coins through touch alone. Again, in each case, cultural exposure to such items (cultural equivalence) is critical for optimal performance.

LURIA NEBRASKA NEUROPSYCHOLOGICAL BATTERY

Luria Nebraska Neuropsychological Battery is designed to assess a broad range of neuropsychological functions in preadolescent children. It is particularly helpful in planning rehabilitative programs. The Receptive Speech subtest measures the ability to understand spoken speech, comprehend words, and understand simple sentences and grammatical structures. Expressive speech measures fluency and requires the child to repeat words and sentences from memory and engage in spontaneous speech. Reading requires the child to read letters, words, phrases, and sentences. On each of these subtests, the child is expected to know the language in which the test is being assessed, and as such, linguistically diverse children are at a disadvantage (Fox, 1991). The bio-cultural assessment system, via its second tier, recommends contextualizing words in a sentence, and this may prove beneficial on these tests as well.

In a similar manner, the Arithmetic test on the Luria could allow use of paper and pencil as is recommended on the second tier of the bio-cultural assessment system instead of the present standard form in which the child is required to perform tasks mentally. Intellectual Processes subtest, which requires a child to identify the similarities and differences between two things, again assumes that the children may have been exposed to the objects in the first place in order to understand the commonalities and differences. The bio-cultural assessment system allows the examiner to substitute the objects for those more in keeping with the child's cultural experiences (cultural equivalencies).

RAVEN PROGRESSIVE MATRICES

The Raven Progressive Matrices, which estimates nonverbal cognitive ability, is used in its traditional standard instruction format to assess the enhancement performance of children who had scored poorly, such as poor planners. However, such children tend to show gains when verbalizations are permitted in the dynamic bio-cultural assessment approach as opposed to standard instruction.

Other tests that can be used in neuropsychological assessment are the Three Dimensional Block Construction Test, which requires the child to construct an exact replica of the three block models, a pyramid, an 8-block four-level construction, and a 15-block four-level construction. Again, the second tier of the bio-cultural assessment system that allows for test–teach–retest could be applied here.

The Selective Attention, Expressive test—The Stroop Test (Stroop, 1935), which comprises word reading, could also benefit from the bio-cultural assessment approach, given that the time factor to determine the speed of the reading of the words (speed of personal tempo) could be suspended, as in the second tier of the bio-cultural assessment system.

The points raised in this chapter confirm the position of the authors taken thus far in this book, and that is, caution is needed when considering the diagnostic accuracy in interpreting neuropsychological test data on a child (Ivnik, Smith, Petersen, Boeve, Kokmen, and Tangalos, 2000). Training implications for neuropsychological assessment for school personnel are discussed in Chapter 12.

CHAPTER 9

Personality Assessment and Culturally Diverse Children

The issue of assessing the personality characteristics and emotional functioning of culturally diverse children continues to be a concern, particularly since certain ethnic groups (e.g., African-Americans) are overrepresented in the psychiatric care system and other groups (e.g., Asians) are underrepresented relative to the general population (Rosenblatt and Attkisson, 1992). An important value of assessment is its potential to guide the best intervention possible. It is therefore vital to find ways to ensure that assessment is comprehensive and contextual, rather than limiting and purely symptomatic of a disorder. In order to accomplish this, it is first important to recognize the socio-cultural factors that impede or promote a healthy adjustment to a particular society. Equally critical is the recognition of the limitations of the diagnostic nosology in diagnosing culturally diverse families. The need for cultural consultants to aid in increasing therapists' knowledge, skills and sensitivity should aid in mitigating biases and misdiagnosis (Budman, Lipson and Meleis, 1992).

In order to evaluate the emotional stability of culturally diverse clients, we suggest incorporating several models, namely:

1. The National Institute of Mental Health Culture and Diagnosis Group (Mezzich, Kleinman, and Fabrega, 1993), in which the authors explored issues of culture and psychiatric diagnosis.

2. Herron, Ramirez, Javier and Warner's (1997) Contextual Assessment Approach, in which the authors offered an organizational focus for assessment that can be more reflective of issues facing culturally diverse families.

3. Armour-Thomas and Gopaul-McNicol's (1997, 1998) Bio-Cultural Approach to assessment.

All of these models offer culturally relevant prescriptions, interpreting personality characteristics within the culture-specific living context. In other words, the interaction of the environment and one's maturation is foremost in the assessment process. For example, in many societies it is more acceptable to say "I am feeling nervous" than to say "I am feeling depressed." The patient may really be going through depression, but has not been socialized to view depression as an acceptable form of emotional distress. Furthermore, the culturally acceptable self-designation of nervousness may be the only descriptor the patient knows to describe his/her emotional discomfort.

The assessor ought to be aware also of the latent problem and not only the manifest problem (Herron et al., 1997). This is quite common with culturally diverse families who have been socialized to keep family secrets within the family, sharing with the assessor only what they deem relevant (Gopaul-McNicol, 1993, 1997).

CULTURAL DEFINITION/CULTURAL IDENTITY

Johnson (1988) and Frisby (1992) refer to culture as the beliefs, customs, achievements, language and history of a group of people that are manifested in their behavioral norms. In other words, one's cultural socializations influence his/her cognitions, feelings, self concept, and, ultimately, the diagnostic process. In general, Eastern cultures relate more to a group cultural identity, whereas Western culture relates more to an independent individual cultural identity (Lu, Lim, and Mezzich, 1995). It is vital to know these issues when assessing a child's personality and emotional functioning. Other factors to consider are the child's country of origin and its political development (political unrest), the child's reasons for migration, the child's family values, beliefs, customs, and linguistic competence, as well as his/her attitude about psychotherapy. It is also important to examine any trauma that may have taken place in the child's life so that posttraumatic stress can be assessed, as well as any losses in the child's life, such as disillusions. All of this is impor-

TABLE 1   Personality Assessment with a Culturally Diverse Child

---

1. Migration History
   • Country of origin and its political development (independent, political unrest)
   • Individual, family and community support
   • Individual and family educational level
   • Individual and family socioeconomic status
   • Reasons for migrating
   • Which family members or close friends were left behind
   • Any traumatic experiences prior to migration
2. Financial History
   • Present financial support
   • Previous financial security, material losses
3. Educational/Career Exploration
   • Educational level, educational changes/losses
4. Cultural Norms
   • What is normal/abnormal in the culture of origin
   • What is normal/abnormal in the host culture
5. Concept of Psychotherapy/Mental Illness
   • What does the child and his/her family think about mental illness
   • What does the child and his/her family think about psychotherapeutic services
6. Level of Acculturation/Cultural Identity
   • Pre-encounter stage, transitional stage, transcendent stage
7. Support Systems
   • Family, community, school, churches
8. Differential Diagnosis/Culture-bound Syndromes
   • Attention deficit hyperactive disorder or healthy verve
   • Oppositional defiant disorder or a true response to discrimination
   • Adjustment disorder or depression
   • Posttraumatic stress disorder or depression
   • Schizophrenia or spirit possession or healthy cultural paranoia

---

tant to ascertain if the therapist is going to avoid misconceptions based on cultural stereotypes or even ignorance. Finally, the child's level of acculturation, or cultural identity as termed by Helms (1985), is vital to assess since intercultural interactions influence one's behavior (Gopaul-McNicol, 1993). Helms' three-stage model of cultural identity—the pre-encounter stage whereby the individual is still enmeshed in the Eurocentric worldview, the transitional stage where the individual re-identifies with his/her culture of origin, and the transcendent stage when the individual becomes more bicultural and uses the experiences from both cultural groups that best fit his/her own circumstances—is yet another important dimension in assessing the emotional functioning and personality characteristics of a child. Table 1 gives a cursory view of the critical areas to examine in assessing the personality and emotional functioning of a child.

COMMONLY ACCEPTED PSYCHOPATHOLOGICAL DISORDERS AMONG CULTURALLY DIVERSE CHILDREN

While many disorders are seen in many cultures, the manifestation and acceptance of these disorders are dependent upon the cultural values (Draguns, 1987). In general, mood (except depression) and anxiety disorders are more prevalent and accepted than are personality and thought disorders (Gopaul-McNicol, 1993). In most developing nations, repression of one's desires creates difficulties that are seen in a more psychosomatic manner, such as vague physical aches, pains, dizziness, upset stomach, gas problems (mainly reported in the stomach) and nerves. Often, these psychosomatic complaints are masking a depressive type of disorder that the individual, for cultural reasons, is unable to talk about. The reason is most likely because physical complaints are more accepted than psychological ones because most people around the world have not conceptualized emotional/mental illness in the same manner as Westerners have. The truth is that physical complaints elicit much compassion, whereas psychological complaints result in a sense of weakness and failure, especially on the part of males. Thus, secondary gains are often achieved because the person is relieved of their responsibilities because of these ailments (Gopaul-McNicol and Brice-Baker, 1997). Generally, the stresses are not limited to that of defiant children, but they include spousal abuse, marital tensions, infertility, the death of loved ones, querulous relatives, poverty and the "evil eye" of family or friends. The response is usually in the form of physical and psychological symptoms that result in psychosomatic ailments, such as asthma (very commonly found among inner-city urban children), heart weakness, bodily aches, digestive problems, sleep disturbance and eating disorders. A classic example is captured in the following vignette:

Case Example

> Mary was failing four of seven courses. She tried, to no avail, to explain the situation to her parents. They refused to respond to her concerns that the courses are difficult and instead, they said that she did not try hard enough. Suddenly, she developed many ailments which were diagnosed as nerves. She was given Valium to address the "physical problem." This resulted in complaints of stomach aches, dizziness and the inability to carry out the usual household chores and school assignments. Mary's parents were forced to address these physical ailments and were more sensitive to her academic failings. Mary, through these psychosomatic complaints, got her parents to respond to her needs and to be less harsh on her when she did not pass her courses.

Thus, any cross-cultural study on psychopathological disorders would be aimed at answering the following questions: Can a direct causal relationship be drawn between an individual's culture and his/her symptoms, and if the relationship is not causal, is there some other way in which the culture influences the maintenance and elimination of symptoms? The former question is difficult to answer, because it has always been a compelling task in psychology to state with a high degree of certainty that one variable causes another. When an individual presents himself/herself for a psychological evaluation, the examiner is confronted with many aspects of the latter question. For example, in what way have cultural norms influenced when a child's family decides to seek psychological help? Or, what indigenous approaches exist for dealing with the pathology in question? Before addressing these questions, it is necessary to examine the risk factors that can lead to mental stress.

RISK FACTORS FOR THE DEVELOPMENT OF MENTAL DISORDERS

IMMIGRATION

Risk factors are those variables or situations which have the potential to make an individual or group of individuals vulnerable to developing a particular disorder. One potential source of stress for the culturally diverse client is immigration (Gopaul-McNicol and Brice-Baker, 1998). For some, the very reason for leaving their countries and the means by which they had to leave results in traumatic reactions. The components of stress come from having to flee one's native country because of persecution, often abruptly, possibly with no chance to say goodbye to loved ones, with no opportunity to plan, no means of bringing belongings on the trip and living in constant fear of discovery.

Another considerable source of stress for immigrant children, regardless of their reason for migration, is leaving family members behind. Sometimes anxiety symptoms are not even present until after the family is reunited. Having lived through separation in the past makes any future separation, real or imagined, a very toxic issue (Brice, 1982). Once an entire family or individual has successfully left, and the immigrant has established connections in the United States, such as securing a home, other risk factors must be considered during evaluation and therapy. Adjustment disorder with anxious mood is a consideration when assessing reactions to a new home, a new physical environment, strange foods, and unfamiliar and brutally cold weather.

Dressler (1985) has posited another risk factor for stress associated with immigrant status. He suggests that the immigrant child's exposure to the American or Western lifestyle without adequate means to access that lifestyle can make one vulnerable for the development of symptoms. In his study, he tests the hypothesis that the greater the gap between the lifestyle the immigrant is exposed to and the immigrant's ability to attain that lifestyle, the high-

er the level of belief in other explanations such as witchcraft and the super-
natural. His hypothesis was supported empirically in two of the three groups
he examined.

FAMILY ROLE CHANGES

Unlike in Western societies, such as the United States, where nuclear families
operate independently (Saeki and Borow, 1987; Sue and Zane, 1987; Triandis,
1987), among many immigrant families, the nuclear family is part of the
extended family. To a large extent, relationships with neighbors, institutions
such as the church and the school are perceived in a collective, family-like
manner, rather than in individualistic terms (Triandis, 1987; Thrasher and
Anderson, 1988; Gopaul-McNicol, 1993). Likewise, whereas in Western societies egalitarian structures of power are nurtured and individualistic pursuit of
happiness and fulfillment are emphasized (Kim, 1985; Sloan, 1990; Gushue
and Sciarra, 1995), among immigrants, individual desires are suppressed for
those of the family and even for the society. In many developing nations, relationships are hierarchical and power is dependent upon age and gender
(Gopaul-McNicol, 1993, 1997). Parents and elders are well respected in these
societies, unlike in the North America, where youth takes precedence over the
aged. Loyalty and respect for one's elders are emphasized to the extent that it
is disrespectful to discuss negative feelings about one's parents to a stranger.
Moreover, children are socialized to have a relational value community-type
orientation with a focus more on societal commitment than individual development (Brice, 1982; Gopaul-McNicol and Brice-Baker, 1997). So an individual who pursues his/her own personal interest and forsakes the family's goals
is perceived as self-centered and avaricious. Thus, the self is defined more with
respect to the roles the individual plays in the community and the family and
is less conceived in individualistic terms. Because of this modus operandi,
interpersonal and intrafamilial boundaries are not as clearly defined as they are
in North America and the need for privacy is seen as selfish.

Family therapists often get referrals when the family has been reunited.
Such reunification calls into question family roles and family loyalty. Minuchin
(1974) has stressed the importance of maintaining optimal family structure.
Every family has a structure which provides family members with a blueprint
for how to behave and knowledge of what is expected of them. It specifies gender roles (male and female) and generational roles (grandparents, parents, and
children). Minuchin and other structural family therapists contend that when
a structure is altered (i.e., boundaries between generations get blurred or
members of one generation assume the duties of another generation), it gives
rise to anxiety in the family. The precipitator for the change in structure, the
gradualness or abruptness of the change and the family's accommodation to it

are just some of the factors which may influence who becomes the symptom carrier (the family member who develops a clinical disorder).

RACISM

Another risk factor is the experience of racism (Brice-Baker, 1996; Gopaul-McNicol, 1993; Gopaul-McNicol and Brice-Baker, 1997). Racial discrimination is something that immigrant families have difficulty negotiating at times, and it is something they have in common with African-Americans. However, there are some differences; immigrant people of color usually tend to be in the racial majority in their countries of origin. They did not experience the lynching, the hosings or the Jim Crow laws that characterized the Black experience in the United States. What both groups have experienced is a definition of who is Black which has been imposed on them by Whites (Gopaul-McNicol, 1993). In the immigrant, considerable emphasis is placed on skin color because one's "degree of browness" has been so inextricably linked to social class. It is shocking for the immigrant on the lighter end of the color continuum to come to the United States and be "relegated" to the lowest rung of society. Anxiety can run high when one realizes that the lighter shade of his/her skin will not afford him/her any protection from discrimination.

DIFFERENTIAL DIAGNOSIS AND CULTUROLOGICAL ISSUES IN PERSONALITY ASSESSMENT

While there is an incredible body of literature on the topic of psychopathology among people of African-American ancestry, considerably less literature exists on its cross-cultural manifestations. In the mental hospitals, anxiety has been reported as the most frequent complaint among children and adolescents and depression has been noted as the second most commonly diagnosed psychopathology (Kashani et al., 1987). However an intriguing paradox between immigrant status and mental health has been raised; although immigrants tend to report a high number of symptoms of psychological distress, when prevalence of psychiatric disorders are examined, immigrants tend to show lower rates of mental health difficulties than their U.S.-born counterparts (Burnam et al., 1987). Evidently, these apparently disparate findings raise concerns about the validity of westernized diagnostic criteria for immigrants as a group. The Diagnostic and Statistical Manual of Mental Disorders – III-R, like its predecessors, assumes that across cultures and across populations, people manifest psychiatric distress similarly. However evidence from cross-cultural studies of depression and other mental disorders suggest otherwise (Marsella et al., 1973;

Tseng et al., 1986). The DSM-IV, unlike its predecessors, attempted to address specific cultural factors endemic to cross-cultural populations.

There is no question that cultural factors play an important role in personality assessment. This is because in assessing the emotional adjustment of immigrant children, it is necessary to examine the normal acculturation problems that any immigrant child can experience upon entry into the United States. In making a healthy adjustment to a new environment, immigrants will first tend to draw on their cultural background as a form of reference in the same way that kindergarten students draw on their home experiences. Many immigrant children, when they first arrive, are readjusting to their parents after several years of separation, since children are often initially left behind with relatives while the parents get settled and established in the host country. During this period, children become quite attached to their caretakers whom they come to know as their parents. When these children are reunited with their natural parents, conflicts arise around such issues as family relations, discipline and culture. Conflicts also emerge when children are at different adaptation phases from their parents. Immigrant children can face overwhelming problems in school as they contend with the cultural clash between the norms of their country and the expectations in the host country (Goodstein, 1990). In addition, immigrants typically come from homogeneous nations; they are accustomed neither to racial and ethnic diversity nor to the flagrant racism found in the United States. It is, therefore, common for them to experience confusion and cultural conflict. As a general practice, mental health workers ought to conduct culurological assessment of immigrant clients to avoid misdiagnosis.

Several areas of misdiagnoses can result because of these cultural clashes. Anxiety disorders, in particular posttraumatic stress disorder, depression and schizophrenia, are the most commonly found misdiagnoses (Gopaul-McNicol, 1993) and therefore, as with the previous chapters, we will attempt to address in this chapter the major areas of mental disorders where culturally diverse clients are mis-assessed as having emotional problems. A more culurological approach is examined as psychopathological symptoms/syndromes are judged by clinicians vis-à-vis an understanding/knowledge of the cultural norms of the client's cultural identity.

CHILDHOOD DISRUPTIVE DISORDERS:

Attention Deficit Hyperactive Disorder (ADHD) or Healthy Cultural Verve

The essential features of ADHD and its diagnostic criteria are outlined in DSM-IV. Cultural-specific factors are commonly noted among ethnic and culturally diverse children. Allen and Boykin (1992) discussed how the Afro-cultural dimension of verve (preference for high levels of variable and intense stimulation) are characteristic of the homes of many African-American children. This high sensate stimulation, which arises from doing several things simultaneously—watching television, listening to music (Young and Bagley, 1979), have led to the cultivation of a special receptiveness to heightened variability and intensity of stimulation or high levels of psychological verve. In general, Boykin (1979) found that Black low-income children perform significantly better with greater variability context than with lesser variability context. Hence, the socio-cultural contexts in which these children were nurtured were found to be linked to their emotional and cognitive functioning. Boykin and Allen (1988) noted that the movement expressive orientation typically found in African-American homes and their communities allowed for greater performance and more motivation when cognitive tasks were paired with percussive music or hand-clapping. This does not mean that the present authors and even Boykin and Allen (1988) are proposing that African-American children can only be emotionally and cognitively disciplined if they are exposed to high sensate stimulating situations, but rather, we are attempting to demonstrate that before diagnosing a child as hyperactive, it is necessary to examine his/her cultural upbringing. It is highly possible that what the mainstream society sees as hyperactive is really another culture's ability to perform several things simultaneously—a strength that ought to be valued and not depreciated and labeled negatively. In other words, the present learning context is more congruent with one type of sociocultural ethos than with the other.

Oppositional Defiant Disorder or a True Response to Discrimination

In our clinical work with children, we hear frequent outbursts such as "I have to stand up to the teacher; she is discriminating against me," "I am not defiant; he treats me as if I am stupid because I am not fluent in English, so I will not listen to him." It was clear to us that while some children may appear oppositionally defiant in the classroom, they are quite compliant and conciliatory in other settings where they do not experience a sense of disrespect. These statements were often said and experienced by ethnically, culturally and linguistically diverse children who encountered discrimination by their teachers and other school authorities. Many children who wear the Rastafarian dreadlocks often complain about being persecuted by their teachers, who openly comment on the untidiness of their hair or question why they wear a hat to school, even though the Jewish boy is allowed to wear the yarmulka on his head. These acts of discrimination or perceived unfairness/double standards lead to a self-defense response which is termed oppositional, defiant or outright indolent by the authority figure, resulting in a biased diagnosis of oppositional defiant disorder.

By using the bio-cultural model, we recommend that the child be observed in several settings—home, community and classroom—with another teacher who is more culturally sensitive to the child's cultural practices. This affords us an opportunity to ascertain how the child interacts with others and whether he/she is more receptive to other authority figures.

ANXIETY DISORDERS AND MOOD DISORDERS

Adjustment Disorder or Depression?

Recently, there has been an increase in referrals of immigrant children due to the "depression" noted by school psychologists. While it is important to be concerned about such symptoms as a lack of interest in social activities, feelings of worthlessness, and depressed mood, it is equally important to bear in mind the DSM-IV criteria for a diagnosis of depression and the stages of acculturation that immigrant children go through. Many culturally diverse children who are referred by the school for therapy because of depressed mood are quite social at home and in their communities. In most countries around the world, children are taught to be quiet in the classroom; North American school officials often misinterpret their respect for the classroom setting as withdrawal, shyness, depression, and so forth. Many children say that they are amazed at the liberties that are accorded children in the American classroom. It takes time for them to get used to this liberal, unstructured approach. The bio-cultural model recommends that the examiner simply observe the children on the playground since this should aid in ruling out shyness and withdrawal. A more appropriate diagnosis might be adjustment disorder with depressed mood, since many of these children do not continue to show signs of "withdrawal" for more than 6 months. (According to the DSM-IV, an adjustment disorder cannot have a duration of more than 6 months.) With such clients, unlike those with more serious depression, the experience is transient and suicidal ideation (if it exists at all) is likely to be anxiety-producing. Helping the client cope with the anxieties and practical recommendations for dealing with life in the United States tend to have good results without resorting to pharmacological treatment. In addition, reassuring clients that their symptoms are probably transient and that therapist and the client together can alleviate them will be useful.

Posttraumatic Stress Disorder or Depression/Emotional Disturbance?

Due to natural disasters, such as hurricanes, and ongoing political unrest in many "third world" countries, many children enter the United States traumatized. Thomas (1991) has discussed the responses to trauma given the ages of children. In summarizing the literature, she stated that "the intrusion of memories and thoughts connected to the traumatic event can cause the child to be distracted from an academic task." (p. 5). Ronstrom (1989) found that some children become hysterical at the sound of loud noises. Compounding the already stressful process of migration, these children are faced with memories of violence and death. The behaviors exhibited by children in reaction to these stressors can range from withdrawal to aggression.

Mollica, Wyshak, and Lowelle (1987) emphasized that in spite of the profound stress that these traumatized victims experienced, they have difficulty articulating their trauma-related symptoms, because the expression of these trauma-related symptoms can significantly increase their emotional distress. The result can be withdrawal, deep sadness, poor academic work, behavioral problems in school, and continued difficulty in acculturation. Unfortunately, these behaviors can be misdiagnosed as a form of emotional disturbance or depression. It is vital that the psychologists allow children the time to acculturate and assist in directing families to supportive centers, where they can receive educational and psychological services to aid in the cultural transition.

Social Phobia or Cultural Expectation

In many cultures around the world, children are not expected to speak or socially express themselves in front of adults. Several of our Asian families often commented on how their children are described as withdrawn and shy in the classroom. The families explain the deep-seated cultural practice that children are not permitted to maintain eye-to-eye contact with an adult or to be assertive in the classroom or to speak about dating and sex in the presence of an adult. Therefore, before giving the diagnosis of social phobia, the bio-cultural model suggests allowing for an opportunity for the child to socialize in a setting with his/her peers and not only with adults. Likewise, there must be evidence of social interaction with individuals who are culturally and linguistically familiar. In our practice, we have encountered many children who are termed socially phobic by a therapist, and yet they become quite loquacious when they are socializing with people from similar cultural and linguistic backgrounds. This same scenario is found among women from many parts of the world. Women are, by far, more socially comfortable in the presence of other women than in the presence of men. As such, a diagnosis of social phobia for a woman must take into consideration whether the client is in the presence of her male counterparts who are accorded more deference and given a higher status than their female contemporaries (Gopaul-McNicol, 1993, 1997). In general, it is important to note that some cultures foster and nurture a strong interdependence and reverence between children and adults and between women and men.

Linguistic Limitation or Social Phobia

When assessing the emotional functioning of bilingual children, before concluding that they are fearful of speaking or socializing with their peers, it is important to consider the possibility that limited language proficiency may be a contributing factor to their limited communication skills. Children have often expressed that they are conscious of making grammatical errors, especially in the presence of their classmates. Often, they opt to be silent and listen, thereby sharpening their receptive language skills as they slowly build their expressive language skills, which tend to develop at a slower rate than receptive language development. Thus, a language examination to determine the level of language proficiency in English is needed before concluding that such children are withdrawn, socially phobic and shy.

Thought Disorders

Religious Belief—Spirit Possession or Schizophrenia

In attempting to understand the causes of mental illness, many immigrants, especially those from Eastern cultures, rarely invoke psychological explanations. On the contrary, mental illness is attributed to some form of spiritual restlessness meted out to the individual via a vengeful spirit. Many cultures have a belief in some form of witchcraft that can be worked on someone by an enemy to cause various forms of harm, usually out of envy or to take revenge. Folk belief says that when a person is "possessed," a spirit enters the individual's body, such that the behavior of the person becomes the behavior of the spirit. It is felt that the more suggestible a person is, the more likely he or she is to become "possessed."

Philippe and Romain (1979) found females are more likely than males to become "possessed." These folk beliefs are deeply embedded in the culture and can exert a profound influence on people's lives. Many children in the school system wear a guard, receive spiritual baths (herbal bath with holy water), and have a priest or minister bless the homes, or even throw salt around the house to protect themselves from these evil forces. These beliefs are accepted by most sectors of society, transcending race, class, age and gender. Over the past fifteen years, we have seen several of our clients go to a spiritist while simultaneously seeking psychological help. For example, a woman had sought therapy because her sons had suddenly begun to misbehave "as soon as my mother-in-law had moved into the house." Since her mother-in-law had never accepted her, she attributed the children's misbehavior to her mother-in-law's "evil eye." She talked openly about her suspicions, assuming that the therapist not only understood but would be able to help her in exorcising the children. When the role of a psychologist was explained to her, she was very disappointed that the therapist would not even be able to accompany her to the spiritist. She felt that the problem with her sons was not a psychological one, but a spiritual one. Given the intensity of her belief, and in keeping with the bio-cultural model, it was recommended that she seek the counsel of a spiritist first and then resume therapy after if the negative behaviors of her sons continued after the "bad spirits" were removed from them. She was receptive to this idea and more trusting of the psychological treatment process after she had taken the children to the spiritual healer.

Thus, a diagnostician/therapist who hears a parent say, "My child is not conforming because an evil spirit is on him" and then sees the child wearing a chain with a big cross (guard) should neither be alarmed nor think that the family is weird. Similarly, when a woman attributes her husband's infidelity or lack of familial interest to the fact that "someone gave him something to eat that has him tottlebey [stupid]," she is not imagining something, but is expressing a cultural assessment of her husband's behavior.

The individual who says, "I see the evil spirit in my house" or "The evil spirit talked to me," is not necessarily hallucinating, nor is the individual who says "God came to me and told me to give up my job, so I did" necessarily delusional. If mental health professionals are not aware of the folk system, they may misdiagnose a client or devalue or demean folk culturological behaviors. The major point for therapists in assessing psychiatric problems in immigrant families is to try to determine the difference between "being possessed" and true mental illness. When dealing with immigrants, the area of most confusion is in the accurate assessment of schizophrenia, particularly paranoid schizophrenia.

To make a differential diagnosis, it is first necessary to do a thorough historical assessment of the individual's psychosocial, behavioral, and cognitive functioning. Schizophrenics often exhibit dysfunctions in thought, form, perceptions, affect, sense of self, interpersonal functioning, and psychomotor behavior. To be given a diagnosis of schizophrenia, at least two of the following elements must have existed for at least 6 months: delusions, hallucinations, incoherence or marked loosening of associations, catatonic behavior or flat or grossly inappropriate affect. In addition, functioning in such areas as work, self-care, and social relations must be markedly low. Lefley (1979) found that the responses of "possessed" victims reflected little of the impulsiveness, lability and free-flowing emotionality which characterize schizophrenia. In fact, while "their consciousness is altered, it is not dissociated in the form of a split personality," as is commonly seen with schizophrenics (Lefley, 1979). Schizophrenia is generally treated with antipsychotic drugs, which are useful for eliminating the delusions and hallucinations and alleviating thought disorder.

Another issue is that many immigrants, while acculturating, may exhibit psychotic symptoms due to situational stress. Regarding the folk beliefs, it is enough to say that it is a pattern of social behavior which has been learned (by constant exposure from childhood onward) and in which people have been conditioned to believe. In other words, it is culturally sanctioned and may even be considered a spiritually uplifting experience. "Possession is not abnormal, it is normal" (Wittkower, 1964). For people who endorse the spiritual unrest view, the duration can range from one day to several years. The major point is that many people from culturally diverse backgrounds believe a spiritist can remove the evil spirit and free the individual from this "evil force." Therefore, whereas schizophrenics have difficulty eradicating the psychosis, the "possessed" ought not.

Schizophrenia or Healthy Cultural Paranoia

Grier and Cobbs (1968) and Boyd-Franklin (1989) spoke of the "healthy cultural paranoia" (p. 19) that is typically noted among Black families. This form of suspicion often leads to an extreme cautiousness, which is interpreted by therapists as paranoia. Boyd-Franklin (1989) suggests that this type of response should not be interpreted as pathological or as indicative of needing treatment, since over generations Black families have developed such responses to address the obvious racist, oppressive and discriminatory systems that exist to this day. They have often responded to this oppression by refusing to comply with, trust or identify with persons who differ from themselves.

Schizophrenia or Language Disorder

If the assessment is conducted in a language other than the individual's primary/first language, the therapist has to be cautious that alogia is not because of linguistic impediments. Many culturally diverse children who speak a language that differs from their native language tend to become impatient, sometimes withdrawn, non-communicative and may even manifest a loosening of associated thoughts as they move from one language to the other. This loosening of association, coupled with the frustration of not being able to articulate freely what they feel, may give the child an appearance similar to schizophrenics whose speech is disorganized and incoherent and whose affect is flat.

THE RELEVANCE OF SOME COMMONLY USED TESTS WITH CULTURALLY DIVERSE POPULATIONS

OBJECTIVE ASSESSMENT OF PERSONALITY—THE MMPI-2

The Minnesota Multiphasic Personality Inventory - 2 (MMPI) is commonly used by mental health workers to assess the emotional and mental functioning of culturally diverse clients, particularly in clinical and mental health hospital settings (Duckworth and Anderson, 1995). It is popular among mental health clinicians for several reasons: (a) it is relatively easy to administer and score; (b) it is an objective psychodiagnostic measure; (c) it contains new validity, content and supplemental scales, as well as an abundance of correlate and interpretive data, which are useful with ethnic minority populations (Velasquez, Gonzales, Butcher, Castillo-Canez, Apodaca and Chavira, 1997).

Butcher and Graham (1994) and Velasquez et al. (1997) suggest using the MMPI-2 and not the MMPI with Chicano clients since there are less chances of over-pathologization of Chicanos. Given our clinical experiences with both measures with African-American, Latino, Haitian and English-speaking Caribbean clients, we are in agreement with these authors. We also recommend administering all of the questions and not "cutting corners" by only administering the basic clinical and validity scales since this can lead to "faulty or invalid conclusions" (Velasquez et al., 1997).

Given the lengthiness of the MMPI-2, it is important to ascertain the educational level of the client and his/her ability to read English or understand the questions being addressed to him/her. It is important to note that children have a tendency to "code switch" as they move between languages, depending on the profundity or intensity of the issues being discussed. In many ways, this can complicate the assessment process, since the question now becomes in which language does the client display more/less pathology. Like Velasquez et al. (1997), we believe that language can mediate or help express psychopathology. As such, mental health workers should be aware that a client may have a distinctly different profile in one language versus another. The best way to determine which language to assess the child in is to ask the him/her about his/her language proficiency (which language can the child read and write better in) and language dominance (in which language does the child feel more comfortable disclosing his/her feelings or discussing emotional issues).

Interpretation is yet another issue with the use of the MMPI-2. Mental health workers should always look at the sociocultural context of the client to examine the notion of functional equivalence of diagnostic categories across cultures (Jones, 1978; Jones and Zoppel, 1979; Jones and Korchin, 1982); this involves the client's beliefs about which behaviors are functional and which behaviors are dysfunctional, what is the client's cultural expression of psychopathology, and the points raised on culturally competent assessment in Chapter 3. Mental health workers must be mindful of stereotypes such as "all Latino males are macho" or "all Black women are aggressive." In general, before making any interpretation, the bio-cultural model recommends that the examiner use other tools, such as observations in settings beyond the testing situation. In other words, a more cultural approach to assessment, interpretation, diagnosis and treatment is strongly suggested.

PROJECTIVE ASSESSMENT OF
PERSONALITY—THE TAT

From a psychometric perspective, it is very difficult to develop standardized projective tests due to reliability and validity factors (Holtzman, 1980; Javier & Herron, 1998). Transforming the test into objective scores further complicates the problem because of the imposition of arbitrary categories of response types (Snowden and Todman, 1982).

The major criticisms of projective tests are their culture-bound stimuli and culture-bound interpretations. One such criticism is the lack of stimulus familiarity (stimuli not being psychologically meaningful to ethnic minorities), which limits the respondent's relevant participation. In keeping with the bio-cultural model, we recommend that the examiner look at specific sociocultural familiar situations and their cross-cultural applications when assessing culturally diverse clients. This is critical because certain values, such as achievement, do not have the same conceptual equivalence in all cultural groups. In other words, the same variable may elicit, different behaviors from one cultural group as opposed to another. Further questioning of the child and observation in his/her natural setting would certainly help to contextualize the responses and even parallel Western psychological constructs in another culture.

SOME LIMITATIONS OF THE BIO-CULTURAL
MODEL IN PERSONALITY ASSESSMENT

In general, like all areas of assessment discussed thus far, cross-cultural personality assessment is also difficult to conduct due to its cultural relativity. It is therefore important to validate culturally different responses and culturally different methodology associated with these responses. Concerns such as whether there are clinical requirements for the assessment of the child's emotional functioning are often difficult to answer even with this comprehensive model.

In addition, this model utilizes standardized inventories in its first tier, which can still be misleading if used with non-English-speaking children on whom the tests may not have been standardized. The use of any test with a population for which it was not developed can be completely inappropriate, and any data generated could have the danger of being misinterpreted (Holden, 2000, p. 288).

Moreover, cogent demonstrations of cross-cultural examples of equivalence have not been applied routinely in practice with culturally diverse populations, nor are there any available norms. However, norms for qualitative, informal-type tests are difficult to secure, and this is why the authors have always asked the question, Is the examiner a psychologist or a psychometrician? A psychologist is comfortable relying on his/her clinical skills, observations, informal interviews, unstructured questionnaires, etc. in assessing the psychoeducational functioning of a child. A psychometrician relies on standardized tests only and rarely utilizes his/her clinical skills in a qualitative manner.

Training implications for psychologists and other mental health workers are discussed in more detail in Chapter 12.

CHAPTER 10

Cultural Issues in Vocational/Guidance Assessment

It has been postulated that the profession of vocational evaluation has lost its usefulness and is dying (Parker and Schaller, 1996; Thomas, 1999). With the need for shorter, more cost-productive services, there is a school of thought that the traditional formal comprehensive vocational assessment is outdated and should be replaced by a more informal process that focuses on self-report inventories and interviews (Lustig, Brown, Lott and Larkin, 1998; Lichtenstein, 1993; Thomas, 1999).

After conducting a thorough literature review in the area of vocational assessment, it was clear from the onset that minimal research has been done with culturally and ethnically diverse individuals. The literature seems to conclude that race still accounted for a substantial amount of variance in the performance of individuals who are assessed by the existing standardized vocational assessment measures (Avolio and Waldman, 1994; Blair, Blair and Madamba, 1999; Fouad, Cudeck and Hansen, 1984; Fouad and Hansen, 1987; Montoya and Swanson, 1992). The findings also suggest that standardized tests are still the most commonly used means of assessing the vocational interests of ethnically and culturally diverse families.

Blair, Blair and Madamba (1999) posit that culture-based distinctions across ethnic groups may affect the academic success of minority students. In like manner, the authors have shown that social class-based characteristics are considered the best predictors of academic performance among minority students, and that educational achievement differences across racial groups can be traced back to the familial context. Sue and Okazaki's (1990) notion of relative functionalism assumes that minority students drawing from their respective cultural experiences develop "folk theories" about their likelihood of success. Alva (1993) proposes that students' vocational aspirations rely greatly upon the students' cultural values and practices and the values, practices and conditions of the school.

When cultural or ethnic comparisons are made against a standard defined by the mainstream dominant group, the result usually tends to be prejudicial because of the erroneous assumptions that the measures used can be universally applied. Clearly, the assessment establishment has not been able to foster enough cross-cultural equivalence nor do they understand how denigrating an experience it is for an individual to be given such low-level expectations.

A vignette that may help capture a common experience that non-white students encounter at the college level happened to one of the authors of this book. The primary author in her very first semester at college was told by the guidance counselor (White female) that Blacks do not usually complete a doctorate, so she should reconsider pursuing psychology as a career interest since one is required to have a doctorate to be a clinical psychologist in practice. This counselor really thought she was offering sound advice, which was predicated on her assuming the values, affect and behaviors of the Euro-American mainstream culture. This assumption was the impetus of her counsel and her belief in such Nigrescence theories.

This chapter will examine how vocational counselors often unintentionally direct children into professions based on an IQ score or on a stereotypical version of what is culturally expected of them. Girls often claim that they are guided away from professions such as engineering. Very rarely are motivation, a sense of determination and discipline factored into the advisement. The practice of matching careers to personality patterns through standardized tests, such as the Strong Campbell and the Holland Directed Search, often can lead to misadvisement. In addition, this chapter will discuss how vocational assessment measures, such as the Kuder, Strong Campbell, and Holland Directed Search, may not be the best option for assessing the vocational interest of culturally diverse families. Career exploration and career guidance for children who are not exposed to positive role models will also be examined in keeping with a bio-cultural perspective.

Career development has been defined as the total constellation of psychological, sociological, educational, physical., economic, and chance factors that combine to shape the career of any individual over the life span (Super, 1987).

McKenzie (1986) found that the cultural backgrounds of West Indian-American clients affect their career choices and their biculturalism induces conflict within their families. Since they also have strong taboos against seeking counseling (Gopaul-McNicol, 1993; McKenzie, 1986), vocational counselors must go beyond standardized tests when working with clients across cultures. It is critical to recognize the uniqueness in each culture and not to underemphasize the impact of culture, experience, and exposure in one's career choice and in one's willingness to cooperate on standardized tests of vocational assessment.

Delahunty (1988), Krumboltz (1994), Raskin (1985, 1987), Super (1987, 1992a, 1995a), Super and Sverko (1995), and Westbrook and Sanford (1991) all examined, in different ways, how the values of individuals are expressed differently, depending on the work setting and situation. They also emphasized how it is the influence and interaction of both personal characteristics (such as one's values, skills and abilities) and external/environmental factors (such as the state of the economy) which, when combined, determine one's career path. Thomas (1999) proposed a community-based assessment which focuses on providing realistic, hands-on evaluation opportunities for individuals with severe and multiple disabilities. All of these authors recommend a broad, multidimensional view of career exploration and, as such, represent the most comprehensive extant theoretical statement in the vocational assessment literature.

DIFFERENTIAL DIAGNOSIS TO CONSIDER IN CROSS-CULTURAL VOCATIONAL ASSESSMENT

LINGUISTIC LIMITATION OR LIMITED VOCATIONAL INTEREST

There are numerous aspects of a child's environment which may substantially influence the child's vocational interest. Characteristics such as the language used at home may be influential factors. Therefore, when assessing the vocational interests of bilingual children, before concluding that their interests are limited, it is important to consider the possibility that limited language proficiency may be a contributing factor to their narrow job selection. Children and adolescents who are not fluent in English reading, comprehension or even in receptive English language skills have often responded in a narrow manner to such tests. To assume that they do not have the ability or the interest to pursue other careers is not to recognize the lack of cultural sensitivity when tests are given in a language different from that of the examinee. It must also be remembered that there are few vocational tests that are given in languages other than English. The Holland Self-Directed Search Tests has a Spanish version, but even when it is translated into Spanish, the question content may be lost or may not have the same meaning to the client's native dialectical lexion. Thus, a language examination to determine the level of language proficiency in English is needed before concluding that such examinees are limited in their vocational interests or ability.

GENDER LIMITATIONS OR LIMITED VOCATIONAL INTEREST

In general, the career choices that girls from developing nations around the world make are determined by culture-specific qualities. In most of these countries, the power structure is typically patriarchal rather than egalitarian, with fathers being considered the major authority within the family unit. Male children are accorded more liberty, both socially and professionally. Girls are encouraged to choose professions like nurse, secretary or elementary schoolteacher. One girl captured the gender bias in career selection by the following vignette:

> My father was so angry when I said I wanted to be a doctor because he felt that this would limit my finding a mate. He felt that no man will want me as a spouse because I will be seen as too masculine and too much of a threat, so I was forced to study nursing.

LIMITED VOCATIONAL INTEREST OR LIMITED VOCATIONAL EXPOSURE

First, it must be pointed out that the questions themselves on vocational tests can be quite confusing for a bicultural/bilingual child (Senior, 1997). For example, on the Holland Self-Directed Search (Holland, 1990) (currently the most commonly used vocational test in high schools), the child is expected to circle yes or no to questions on his/her range of interests. An example of such is "take a course in design." Most culturally diverse children will have difficulty understanding the word "design" in this context, even if they enjoy advertising or architectural work. Likewise, some children have difficulty placing in a relevant context the question "edit a magazine or a journal" because in their native lands, there are no journals and magazines but only newspapers. Thus, in addition to the commonly used standardized tests, in keeping with the bio-cultural model, we recommend interpreting the questions or rephrasing the questions for the examinees so that they can place them in a cultural context to fit their realm of experience. For example, we suggest that the counselor rephrase the question to read "edit the newspapers." By doing so, the child is able to correctly interpret the question to fit his cultural realm of educational/social experiences.

It is therefore critical for "culture fair" vocational assessors/examiners to be aware of the questions on each test that may present some difficulty for culturally diverse children and to assist them with each of these questions by engaging in an item equivalency (Helms, 1985; Armour-Thomas and Gopaul-McNicol, 1998) type of approach. Due to cultural differences in syntax and inventory use of unfamiliar names for familiar activities, Senior (1997) suggests dialoguing with the students to guide them to completion.

Senior (1997) observed that in the school system many culturally diverse students are inadequately prepared for college because they are guided to be laborers than into professional-type careers. In keeping with the proposed bio-cultural model, we also recommend exposing the client to a variety of careers in a very personal and practical way. This was found to be most effective for teenagers who were never exposed in their culture of origin to some careers. In our private practice, we encountered children who aspired to be "a numbers man." Many guidance counselors assume when a child says "I want to be like my father" and the father happens to be employed in an unsavory, illicit profession that the child's aspiration is reflective of his or her vocational interest or motivational level or even his/her intellectual functioning; this is a rather erroneous conclusion. In our practice, we have found that children's career choices were often made due to their limited exposure to a variety of professions. Before concluding that the findings on vocational tests are correct, we would always expose the children to a variety of professions by inviting guest speakers of their ethnic and, if possible, cultural backgrounds, at least once per month to our clinic and have them talk to the children about their careers. Afterwards, children would be allowed to visit the job sites and witness first-hand their career interests.

Likewise, we arrange college fairs approximately once per year in our neighboring communities. This is critical, since interests grow out of what an individual is exposed to. Therefore, the more exposure an individual has, the more he/she would make career choices in keeping with those experiences. The important point to keep in mind is that these vocational tests do not simply reflect one's vocational interests, and as such, a vocational counselor ought not to merely guide a student into a profession because of what is reflected on the test. The bio-cultural model conceives assessment as an ongoing, cyclical process and not a linear unidimensional process, which is more characteristic of an evaluation (Gopaul-McNicol, 1993, 1997). In other words, after giving and reviewing the results of the vocational tests, we suggest conducting a second tier of the assessment process—the assessment-pre-intervention phase—in which the client is exposed to various careers outside of his/her experiential realm. This rules out any chance of the client's choosing a particular career based on limited cultural experiences within a limited context. This phase is where children are exposed to careers and professionals. Levinson and Brandt (1997) offered suggestions for counselors to form a career education program which is integrated within the regular education curriculum. After this pre-intervention phase, we then assess the child again (third phase) via the very same vocational tests and often a different profile emerges. At our clinic, many children showed different interests from those which they reflected in the first phase of the assessment process.

In summary, the vocational assessment phases are as follows:

1. vocational test assessment
2. vocational pre-intervention assessment
3. vocational test assessment.

Clearly, what is represented in this chapter is what has been reflected throughout this book and that is, assessment involves several phases, which include standardizing testing, assessing the potential of a client via an item equivalency approach, and the assessment of a child in his or her natural environment.

Questionnaire to Assist in Assessing the Vocational Interests of Culturally Diverse Clients

1. What types of vocational experiences has this client been exposed to within his/her natural environment?
2. What vocational interests are reflected on the standardized tests and are they in keeping with the results of the standardized tests?

After completing this type of comprehensive three-tier assessment, the role of the vocational counselor is expanded to that of a consultant to teachers, workshop leader to the community, etc. The counselor can now provide ongoing exposure to professionals within the community. Likewise, teachers and parents can be offered training as to how to further enhance the intellectual and vocational potential of children.

At this juncture, having discussed all areas of cross-cultural assessment, we suggest that a cross-cultural perspective be adopted both conceptually and methodologically. In other words, a framework for the assessment of all populations should take the form of a psycho-social, biocultural model as discussed in Chapter 4. Such a framework would allow for empirical manifestations of functional and conceptual equivalences whenever such equivalences arise.

POSSIBLE LIMITATIONS OF THE BIO-CULTURAL MODEL TO VOCATIONAL ASSESSMENT

Given the many limitations of traditional standardized vocational tests, the inclusion of this bio-cultural approach in the career assessment process is very positive, for the most part. By juxtaposing Eurocentric worldviews and career options as the ideal, the magnitude of the differences in the perspectives of culturally and ethnically diverse individuals is even more apparent. The need for cultural clinical expertise predicated on cultural sensitivities, knowledge of diagnostic conceptualizations from a model such as the bio-cultural model, is even more acute as we enter a new millennium, where multiculturalism is considered a fourth force in psychology.

The only limitation of this bio-cultural model in vocational assessment is the lack of normative data, a continued criticism from mainstream professionals of the new approaches espoused by culturally diverse examiners, practitioners and researchers alike.

CHAPTER 11

A Bio-Cultural Approach to Report Writing

Proponents of the bio-cultural theory (Ceci, 1990; Armour-Thomas and Gopaul-McNicol, 1998) contend that a more comprehensive theoretical approach, involving the works of Vygotsky (1978), Gardner (1983, 1993), Sternberg (1985), and Feuerstein (1979), is very important in assessing students from linguistically and culturally diverse backgrounds. Before presenting a sample bio-cultural report, it is necessary to explore some issues in assessment/diagnosis and intervention.

DIFFERENTIAL DIAGNOSIS

With culturally different families, it is critical to conduct differential diagnoses for intellectual assessment, educational assessment, visual-motor assessment and personality assessment. Chapters 5–10 can assist the examiner in conducting differential diagnoses. It is important to rule out why it is not one diagnosis versus the other. For example, for educational assessment, in particular with linguistically different children, it is important to examine whether it is a linguistic issue. In other words, does the child have the skill in his/her native language but perhaps not in English? Has the examiner assessed or recommended that the child be assessed in both languages? This would help to rule out whether it is a delay only in English or in both languages.

To conduct a differential diagnosis for visual-motor assessment, one should examine whether it is a cultural matter or a true sign of a neurological/visual-motor disorder? The examiner should rule out why it is not one versus the other. To conduct a differential diagnosis for personality assessment, it is crucial to examine whether the issue is depression, adjustment disorder, post-traumatic stress disorder, or a psychosomatic disorder. Again, it is important to rule out why it is not one versus the other. Examiners should note that with culturally different children, it is important to rule out cultural factors first (e.g., the extra verve of some children), before diagnosing a child as having an attention deficit hyperactive disorder.

RECOMMENDATIONS

One's recommendations should be based on one's diagnostic impressions after a thorough differential diagnosis is completed. Thus, if after doing intellectual potential assessment, the examiner should recommend what he/she believes are the best ways the teacher, parent, or mental health worker can intervene in working with the child. In other words, if teaching via the test–teach–retest method helped, then the examiner should recommend one-on-one teaching for a particular number of sessions. If extending or suspending time helped, then the examiner should recommend that the child be given extra time and more opportunity for practice. If contextualizing words helped, the examiner should recommend that initially, as the child acclimates to the new environment, he/she should be given an opportunity to receive his/her assignment in a surrounding context. If the child was found to do better on paper-and-pencil tasks than on tasks requiring mental computations, then the examiner should recommend that paper-and-pencil assessment be allowed. If the child is found to have other intelligences, the examiner should recommend programs where these can be further enriched.

For achievement assessment, the examiner should recommend specific remedial programs. While initially the child may be found to need the supportive environment of bilingual education, the goal should be to help this child become proficient in English. Self-contained special education classes are not the least restrictive settings. The examiner should therefore explore other settings with other types of supportive programs before placing a child in self-contained special education classes.

With respect to visual-motor assessment, the examiner should note that a neurological evaluation is not needed if the rotations on the Bender were not truly clinical signs. The differential diagnosis should serve as a guide here. For personality assessment, the examiner can recommend the appropriate treatment intervention based on his/her diagnosis. The examiner must, however, pay close attention to cultural issues, such as religion, family beliefs, role of family members, and culturally prescribed ways of interacting.

In general, the examiner should utilize all of the resources in his/her community—church, social/recreational community programs, after-school programs, legal aid, psychotherapeutic programs, etc. In summary, the examiner must be able to assist the School Based Support Team (SBST), the family and the child to develop a course of treatment that would maximize every opportunity for the child to move from his/her actual functioning to his/her potential functioning within a three-year period. In other words, the child should show significant gains after the intervention period in all areas assessed.

A sample case report is presented below to illustrate the bio-cultural assessment system.

GENERAL REMINDERS FOR THE BIO-CULTURAL ASSESSMENT REPORT

1. When reporting the test results, put sections on:
   (a) *Psychometric (Standardized) Assessment*
       Even when the examiner is writing the psychometric section of the report, the report should be qualitative. For instance, describing the child's strengths and weaknesses in the constructs measured by each subtest.
   (b) *Non-Psychometric Standardized Assessment*
   (c) *Ecological/Cultural Assessment*
       In this section, the examiner should report on what he/she observed in the child's ecology—home, community, playground, school.
   (d) *Other Intelligences*
2. After the examiner reports all of his/her findings, a Diagnostic Impression section and an Educational/Clinical Implications section are recommended. In other words, what are the implications of the findings for the individual in the classroom/work, home and community?

A BIO-CULTURAL REPORT

Name: Michael
School: JHS
Grade: 6th
Language: Spanish

Date of Testing: 5/25/95
Date of Birth: 7/23/82
Age: 12 years 10 months

Reason for Referral and Background Information

Michael was referred for an initial evaluation by his teacher due to academic and behavioral difficulties both at school and at home. Michael arrived from Nicaragua in October 1994 at age 12. His parents had migrated to the United States when he was 5 years old. While in Nicaragua, he resided with an aunt and uncle, but had many problems engaging them interpersonally. His relatives in Nicaragua believe that Michael became defiant and oppositional after his mother left Nicaragua because an explanation as to why she had left was never accorded him. There were reports of much aggression and disrespectful behavior both at school and at home. Teacher reports reflect that Michael's maladjustment subsequent to his mother leaving Nicaragua could be a result of feeling rejected and abandoned by her, since these negative behaviors were not seen while his mother resided in Nicaragua.

The social history conducted on 5/16/95 by the school social worker revealed that since Michael arrived in the USA, he has had difficulty sleeping at night. There are reports of his being nervous, afraid and unhappy. His mother is concerned that he may be depressed. Michael lives with his two sisters, ages 10 and 3. According to his mother, there is much sibling rivalry and jealousy on Michael's part.

Test Administered and Tests Results

Wechsler Intelligence Scale for Children - III

Psychometric Assessment	Range
Verbal Scale IQ	Borderline
Performance Scale IQ	Borderline
Full Scale IQ	Borderline

Current Verbal Scale Score	Range	Current Non-Verbal Scale Score	Range
Information	deficient	Picture Completion	low average
Similarities	deficient	Coding	borderline
Arithmetic	low average	Picture Arrangement	low average
Vocabulary	low average	Block Design	low average
Comprehension	deficient	Object Assembly	borderline
Digit Span	average	Mazes	borderline

Wechsler Intelligence Scale for Children - III

Psychometric Potential Assessment	Range
Verbal Scale IQ	low average
Performance Scale IQ	average
Full Scale IQ	low average

Ecological Assessment
Estimated Overall Functioning   low average to average

Other Intelligences Assessment
Bodily Kinesthetic (Soccer)
Artistic (Painting)

Family Support Assessment   Moderately Low

Wide Range Achievement Test-III

	Grade Score	Percentile	Standard Score
Reading	1st	.9	52
Spelling	2nd	2	70
Arithmetic	4th	14	84

Bateria Woodcock Psico-Educativa En Espanol – Revisado

	Grade	Age Equivalent
Reading	4.4	10–4
Math	4.9	10–4
Written Language	3.9	9–6

Vocational Assessment—Interest Determination, Exploration and Assessment System (IDEAS Inventory)

Bender Gestalt Motor Test
   Koppitz Error Score 8
   Age Equivalent – Not Scorable
   Bender Recall – 5 out of 9

Beck Depression Inventory – Clinical Borderline Depression

Vineland Behavior Adaptive Scales – Parent Edition Range
   Communication   Low
   Social   Moderately Low
   Daily Living Scales Adequate

Social History
   Human Figure Drawings
   Tell-Me-A-Story (TEMAS)
   Clinical Interview
   Spanish Inventory
   Parent Interview
   Teacher Questionnaire

Language Dominance
    Vocabulary Subtest   Proficiency Rating
    Spanish Expressive Vocabulary   Low average
    English Expressive Vocabulary   Deficient

Behavioral Observation

Michael, a pleasant, petite young man presented himself in a cooperative, compliant manner. He had a good disposition and was motivated to do all of the tasks assigned to him. Even upon completion of the testing, Michael asked the examiner if he could do more. He was not fatigued and saw these types of tests as reinforcing to him. In general, his response time was slow and he approached the testing in a cautious, reflective manner. When he clearly did not know the answer, he still persisted, but became noticeably frustrated and embarrassed. He would sigh, frown, and seemed upset that he did not know the answer to what he initially perceived as easy. All in all, it was a pleasure testing Michael because he tried hard and was willing to please.

Language Assessment

Michael's language proficiency was tested through the administration of the vocabulary subtest of the WISC-III in both Spanish and English. He is clearly more dominant and more proficient in Spanish. He spoke only in Spanish and requested that the examiner speak only in Spanish. Interestingly, when he engaged in social play with two of his peers after the evaluation, he responded to them in English and they spoke to him only in English. Thus, Michael has some English skills, but is too self-conscious to speak for fear of "saying it wrong." Michael's articulation in English was poor and unclear. On a few occasions, it was necessary to ask him to repeat what he was saying. His English receptive skills were also less developed than his Spanish receptive skills. At this time, since Michael's primary language is Spanish, the supportive environment of a bilingual class is recommended. Such a class would add to his understanding and would enhance learning. Likewise, Michael needs to be evaluated bilingually.
(Listed below each section in italicized writing are more examples of the psycho-cultural model.)

Another Example of Writing a Language Assessment Section

Michael's receptive skills are stronger than his expressive skills, since he had more difficulty expressing verbal ideas than understanding what was said to him. Receptively and expressively, he is more dominant in Spanish, since he responded only in Spanish even when the examiner spoke to him in English.

Of note is that Michael is also more proficient in English since he was better able to perform mathematical computations in English and to read and write in English. He counted up to three in Spanish and knew some of the letters in Spanish. In English, however, he was able to construct sentences and to do applied mathematical problems. It is possible that since he receives instruction in the classroom only in English his English skills far surpass his Spanish skills in spite of his being more socially dominant in his native language. The Spanish translation improved his score in all verbal areas, Michael requires the supportive environment of bilingual instruction and ought to be evaluated bilingually when tested psychologically, educationally and linguistically.

Given the fact that Michael is bilingual and that a Latino/Hispanic population was not used as part of the standardization sample, in keeping with the Chancellor's regulations, the following scores ought to be interpreted with caution and should only be used as a guide for school personnel. The results should be interpreted from both a biological and contextual approach.

TESTS INTERPRETATION

Psychometric Assessment

On the Wechsler Intelligence Scale for Children-III, Michael obtained a full-scale IQ score, which placed him in the borderline range of intelligence. His verbal and nonverbal scores fell in the borderline and low average ranges, respectively.

Subtest analysis indicates considerable subtest variability within both the verbal and nonverbal spheres. In the verbal area (crystallized), Michael was deficient in general information, suggesting that on this psychometric test, Michael is not as alert to the social and cultural factors so typical of American society as measured by the WISC-III. His deficiency in comprehension is also indicative of Michael's limited understanding of the social mores here in the USA as assessed on the WISC-III. Michael was also deficient in verbal abstract reasoning, suggesting that, on this test, Michael has difficulty placing objects and events together in a meaningful group. In arithmetic and vocabulary, Michael was low average. This is indicative of inadequate arithmetic skills on the WISC-III, as well as poor language development and limited word knowledge as defined by the WISC-III. In auditory short-term memory, Michael was average. Therefore, one can expect Michael to be relatively good at rote memory and sequential processing.

In the nonverbal area (fluid intelligence), Michael was low average in identifying essential missing elements from a whole, suggesting delayed visual alertness, visual discrimination and long-term visual memory on the Wechsler scales. In visual integration, Michael was borderline, suggesting limited perceptual skills, poor long-term visual memory and limited constructive ability commensurate to his age peers nationwide on the Wechsler scales. However, Michael was persistent and tried to put the puzzles together. There was a sense that he was unfamiliar with these items. As such, when he was taught how to connect the pieces, he tended to be more relaxed, although he continued to perform poorly. In visual-motor coordination/motor speed, Michael was also borderline, suggesting slow response time, poor visual short-term memory and limited visual acuity. In nonverbal comprehension, Michael was low average, suggesting a delayed ability to anticipate the consequences of his actions, to plan and to organize ahead of time on the WISC-III. In nonverbal abstract reasoning, Michael was also low average, suggesting below-average ability to perceive, analyze and synthesize blocks on the Wechsler scales.

Psychometric Potential Assessment

When Michael was tested to the limits and when he was not placed under time pressure, and too, when item equivalencies were done, his score was improved by six IQ points in the verbal area and five IQ points in the nonverbal area.

Therefore, in the verbal area, when the vocabulary words were contextually determined, that is, when Michael was asked to say the words in a sentence instead of asking the word "migrate" in isolation, Michael went from low average to average. Since vocabulary is the best measure of general intelligence, Michael is of average potential in the verbal area. Likewise, when Michael was allowed to use paper and pencil on the arithmetic subtest, he went from low average to average.

In the nonverbal area, when time was suspended when presented with the puzzles on the Wechsler scales, Michael went from borderline to low average. Similarly, Michael went from low average to average on the Block Design subtest when he was taught (test–teach–retest) to manipulate the blocks. Thus, again, Michael is of average potential in the nonverbal area, since Block Design is the best measure of nonverbal intelligence on the Wechsler scales. Overall, Michael's potential is average in the nonverbal area.

A total increment of nine scale points in the verbal area and nine scale points in the nonverbal area resulted in an overall IQ increment of 11 scale score points, which resulted in Michael falling in the low average range instead of borderline range when standard procedures were followed.

Other Examples of Psychometric Potential Assessment

Example I
On the block design subtests, Michael got the more difficult items correct after he passed his ceiling point or after time limits had been expended. In his native

country, blocks and puzzles are not games commonly played by children. As such, he was never exposed to block building. It seemed as if he was learning as he went along, that lack of familiarity and, ultimately, anxiety may have been why he did not do as well on the earlier items. As a result, two IQ's were tabulated—one following standardization procedures and one tapping his potential as evidenced by summing all points attained even after he had reached his point of discontinuation.

Example 2
When Michael was asked "In what way are an apple and a banana alike?" and he did not know the answer, interestingly, when asked how a "mango and a banana" are alike, he got it correct. The important thing here is that he knew the concept of fruits.

Example 3
Also of note is that while Michael did not know the word "migrate" in isolation, he knew it when used in a sentence. Thus, if contextualized, Michael's word knowledge and ability to express verbal ideas at varying degrees of abstraction were much higher. In the same manner, while Michael was unable to articulate how a wheel and a ball were alike, he was able to draw how they were both alike and then to state that they were both round. It seems as if he had to first conceptualize their similarity via visual stimuli, then to form the concept of sameness, before being able to express the common factor between these two objects. Therefore, it is not that Michael has not conceptualized this relationship, but rather, that he has to go through a longer process in order to retrieve and articulate the similarity of such a concept.

Example 4
Michael was able to respond to questions previously misunderstood or unanswered when Spanish dialectical terminologies were utilized. Thus, while he did not understand the question "why do you recycle paper?," he was able to respond appropriately to "why do you separate paper in a separate garbage can?". Likewise, while Michael did not understand the question "why do games have rules?," he clearly was able to produce a two-point response when asked "why are rules needed to play marbles?" Thus, merely rewording the directions helped with understanding, resulting in an increased performance.

Example 5
In observing (Sternberg's) atomization information process approach (Triarchic Model), when given the opportunity to slowly process nonverbal reasoning tasks by trial and error, the ability to correctly complete the tasks became successively more automatic.

Example 6

When standardization procedures were not followed, Michael's potential demonstrated an eight-point difference. For instance instead of presenting the visual stimuli for five seconds as in the standard procedure, the Gestalt was shown for 10 seconds (15 seconds for more complicated Gestalts), and word or number sentences were slowly repeated. This process allowed for and resulted in the ability to process information, increase concentration, decrease anxiety and correctly respond. This suggests that when given more time to process and practice learned problem-solving skills, he can perform appreciably better.

Example 7

While initially Michael did not understand the block design subtest, when a test–teach–retest technique was used (that is, when he was taught how to build blocks and puzzles other than those used on the Wechsler scales and was then tested again), he was able to correctly synthesize the more difficult items, to correctly strategize and respond to two out of three previously incorrect questions. Thus, with respect to nonverbal abstract reasoning, he is more average than borderline, as was seen when standard procedures were followed. This also shows that Michael is capable of learning various tasks once they are explained and he is given the opportunity to practice the tasks.

Example 8

When Michael was tested to the limits, for instance, when he was not placed under time pressure, and also, when item equivalencies as well as the test–teach–test techniques were implemented, Michael's score went from borderline to low average/average in the verbal area, borderline to average in the nonverbal area and borderline to low average/average in overall intelligence. Likewise, when the vocabulary words were contextually determined, that is, the words being asked in a surrounding context ("Michael migrated to the USA recently," instead of asking the word "migrate" in isolation), Michael went from low average to average. Since vocabulary is the best measure of general intelligence, Michael is of average potential in the verbal area. In the nonverbal area, Michael went from deficient to low average on the Block Design subtest when he was taught (test–teach–retest) to manipulate the sample block. Thus again, Michael is of low average potential in the nonverbal area since Block Design is the best measure of nonverbal intelligence on the Wechsler scales. Overall, Michael's potential intellectual functioning is borderline.

Ecological Assessment

Of note is that Michael had difficulty on the Mazes subtest (borderline). However, when Michael had to direct the examiner to drive him home and the examiner made a wrong turn, Michael was quickly able to maneuver his way out of a rather complex geographic location. He certainly manifested much intelligence as he located the route. He showed good planning ability and good perceptual organization when placed in a real-life situation. His low average to average intellectual ability was indeed evident from an ecological perspective.

More Examples of Ecological Assessment

Observation of the child in various settings, such as on the playground or in his/her community, offers interesting information.

Example 1 – Item Equivalency in the nonverbal area
The Block Design and Object Assembly subtests are highly influenced by the American culture. When Michael was assessed by other more comparable measures, such as building a chair, he was found to be very superior, given the quick and accurate manner in which he executed the task.

Example 2
Although Michael had difficulty putting the puzzles together on the WISC-III, at home Michael had no difficulty dismantling a fan and putting back together in a one-hour period. Thus, when he was exposed to a more familiar stimulus, he was able to integrate parts into a meaningful whole, so very characteristic of the Object Assembly subtest of the Wechsler scales.

Example 3
Likewise, while Michael was unable to name two American coins, he was able to correctly name and identify the *escudo* and the *peso*, two monetary units from Chile.
   When Michael was asked to perform skills comparable to the puzzles on the Wechsler scales, he went from borderline to average.

Example 4
In the same manner, while Michael did not know who discovered America or who Christopher Columbus was, he knew that Pedro De Valdivia founded Santiago. Thus, if given time to acclimate to this society, it is expected that Michael will learn American history and concepts, resulting in a higher intellectual functioning score.

Other Intelligences Assessment

Michael is described as very athletic, in particular, in soccer. In spite of his small frame, his mother feels that he has a well-developed sense of timing, coordination and rhythm when it pertains to playing soccer. Thus, with respect to his bodily intellectual ability, he seems to be average to above average in his ability to play soccer.

Michael also has an affinity to drawing/painting. He was able to do cartoonlike drawings. His teacher mentioned that he was the best student in his class in art and art-related fields, such as designing things.

More Examples of Other Intelligences Assessment

Example 1 – Musical intelligence

In spite of Michael's deficiencies in the verbal area, he is able to formulate melodic, rhythmic and harmonic images into elaborate ideas, although he never studied music. For instance, he plays the steel pan, the piano, and the *cuatro* without sheet music and with fluency. He also composes music so creatively that in the realm of musical intelligence, he would be considered superior intellectually.

Example 2

According to Michael's parents, he is very musical and plays the guitar for various Hispanic events.

Example 3 - Bodily–kinesthetic intelligence

Michael is able to dance energetically. His dances allow one an opportunity to observe his bodily intelligence in its purest form, with flexibility and high technical proficiency. He is indeed of superior ability in this area.

Example 4

Michael is athletic and excels in grace, power, speed, accuracy and teamwork. His ability to pitch the ball shows his analytic power and resourcefulness. Also noted was his ability to remain poised under great pressure. A well-developed sense of timing, coordination and rhythm results in his being well-executed and powerful in his gross and fine motor motions. His bodily intellectual strength is superior.

Example 5

Michael has an adequate amount of social competence to deal with issues in his community. For instance, he knows which areas in his neighborhood are drug-infested, and how to avoid going there. He repeatedly said, "Here is where the drug people hang out, so don't go there." He also knew that it was unsafe to flash money around and cautioned the examiner about opening her wallet, even in the supermarket.

Visual-Motor Assessment

The borderline performance noted in visual-motor coordination on the Wechsler scales was also seen on the unstructured Bender test of visual-motor coordination. Michael's performance was severely delayed due to seven errors of rotation and one error of integration. Interestingly, when he was asked if his designs were like the examiner's, he quickly gave a negative retort and drew them correctly when asked to draw his exactly like the examiner's. It seems that Michael had difficulties in the conceptualization of the visual impressions and not in the visual perception itself. Thus, he only perceived the Gestalten incorrectly and therefore interpreted them in a concrete way, to fit his realm of experience at this time. Clearly, cultural factors were operating which impeded Michael from responding correctly to the stimuli cards.

Achievement Testing

Michael was found to be on a 4th-grade level in Spanish reading, but a first-grade level in English reading. In math, he was on a 4th-grade level in both English and Spanish. In spelling, Michael was on a 3rd-grade level in Spanish and a 2nd-grade level in English. Thus, he is delayed in his native language in all areas, but is severely delayed in English. Because he has only been residing in the USA for seven months, it is expected that his English skills are going to be limited. With respect to his limited Spanish skills, it must be reiterated that Michael had not been attending school for two years in Nicaragua when he was expelled from school at age ten. Thus, in effect, Michael received education up to a 4th-grade level in his native country. His skills are therefore commensurate with his actual educational experiences. Therefore, this child's prognosis for functioning at a higher educational level is good if he receives intensive instruction in all academic areas.

Vocational Assessment

Michael's scores on the IDEAS Inventory, the other intelligences questionnaire and the clinical interview point to areas of arts and crafts, which he finds most enjoyable and in which he may find the greatest satisfaction. He enjoys making pottery, painting, and is said to be very artistic in his ability to draw pictures of people, places and scenery. Given Michael's intellectual potential and achievement functioning, his professional interest is commensurate to ability. However, career awareness and career exploration are needed as Michael moves on to the high school.

More Examples of Vocational Assessment

Example 1
Michael expressed a desire to become a carpenter or a construction worker. He seems to know much of the trade, and says that he likes to work with wood, likes to help his uncle install doors, windows, and cabinets and molding. He stated that while residing in Nicaragua, on several occasions, he watched the complete building of a house. It was clear to the examiner that he has had exposure to construction-type work in his native country. Career guidance is needed in this area. Furthermore, it would be most beneficial to infuse a motivating factor in Michael's high school career. For instance, work study or after-school projects, such as part time apprenticeships, would serve to mitigate some of the apathy seen during this evaluation. This is important for Michael, who sees himself as much a student as an employee. Math skills of the classroom can be related to the math skills necessary to work with blueprints. Listening to instructions in the classroom can be related to working from the instructions of his supervisors in relation to a layout or in relation to local building codes and their dictates.

Example 2
Michael should review the Occupational Outlook Handbook and get a clear picture of the present and future prerequisites and criteria which he must attain in order to become a construction worker, enter the military, or have access to government jobs. He should also be taught how to be self-employed through the private sector.

Example 3
Michael should also be taught how to acquire and develop interpersonal and intrapersonal communication skills, which are essential to, or indirectly related to, a job situation. The starting point for this exercise would be the development of interview skills, as can be practiced in role-modeling situations. Understanding of how people's personalities vary and affect their working with others should be demonstrated, observed and discussed in relation to Michael's peers, teachers, siblings, parents and employers.

Example 4
Classroom and counseling activities should include writing a business letter, such as those used in draft application letters and letters of inquiry. Moreover, how to prepare a personal data sheet would be another important activity. Vocational counseling, career guidance and career exploration will all be beneficial at this time.

Example 5
Michael would like to become a carpenter. Although he knows little of this trade, he expressed that he enjoys building houses and installing windows and

cabinets. It was obvious during the clinical interview that he needs some vocational exploration. Areas that should be explored with Michael are requirements for his vocational interests, comfort needs, etc. He should be taught how to relate math skills as a carpenter to working with blueprints.

Personality Assessment

The personality tests, the clinical interview and parental interview depict Michael's adjustment as variable. On the one hand, he is a pleasant, charming, delightful, motivated and sensitive youngster. He is interested in learning and wants to be a police officer. These positive behaviors are seen mainly in a one-on-one type situation. On the other hand, the personality tests and the teacher behavior checklist reveal a young man who is angry and relates aggressively to his peers. Michael has reportedly hit, pushed and physically attacked his classmates. He has few friends in class with whom he is able to engage interpersonally. Even children who are from similar cultural backgrounds have difficulty interacting with him. These behaviors were also noted in his native country, leading to his eventual dismissal from school at the age of ten.

Michael also expressed anger to the examiner as he recounted being abandoned by his mother for five years as she immigrated to the USA. He is resentful that he was left behind, even though his sister was left back with him. He is intensely jealous of his younger sisters and feels that he is not as loved as they are. The clinical borderline depression score noted on the Beck does not indicate that he is clinically depressed as such, but that he has turned his anger inward and is experiencing psychosomatic ailments, such as headaches and sleep disturbance. The underlying issue is one of much frustration, anger and insecurity with respect to being loved and the desire on his part to receive more nurturing from his mother and stepfather. He has little communication with his stepfather and there is much guilt on his mother's part with respect to leaving him in Nicaragua. These issues on the part of both mother and son ought to be resolved in family counseling. Family support is moderately low since Michael's mother was not formally educated herself, and does not seem to know how to assist Michael as he acclimates to this society. Family counseling should also empower the family by referring them to community support systems such as a church or an after-school program so that the family will be assisted in their acculturation process. Individual counseling should also focus on building Michael self-esteem, building his self-confidence and coping with being different in his physical appearance. Michael is physically smaller than his male counterparts, and this also affects his self-image. Anxiety reduction training with respect to failing and being "not as smart" should also be provided via counseling.

Other Examples of Writing Personality Assessment

Example 1
The stories elicited from the TEMAS indicate that Michael's aspirations seem to center around survival themes and being able to cope with feelings of anger and fear. His style of relating to his peers is poor, perhaps a reflection of poor opportunities to socialize and/or inability to effectively express his feelings and needs.

Example 2
The current assessment also indicates that one major drawback to Michael's process of learning is his tendency to periodically withdraw and tune out. He is also likely to be highly distractible by both inner and outer stimuli. This tendency to withdraw precludes his concentrating and paying attention, making it difficult for him to benefit from the instruction that is presented.

Family Assessment as Part of Personality Assessment

This brings to the assessment robust knowledge of the family dynamics of the child. Therefore, parenting, child-rearing practices, disciplinary measures, punishments/reinforcers, the language spoken at home, religious values, its relationship to the society at large, as well as its impact on the child, are indeed rich sources of knowledge for school psychologists.

Educational Implications

Michael is delayed in general information, comprehension, vocabulary, arithmetic and verbal abstract reasoning. As a result, remediation should focus on exposure to a broad range of everyday facts, practical reasoning in social situations and word building. Michael should be encouraged to read American literature or the newspaper on a daily basis, to gain more insight of world events and the mainstream cultural views and to help improve in general information. Other resources are the museums, educational television shows, tapes and film documentaries. Teaching same/different concepts should aid in improving verbal abstract reasoning. In addition, vocabulary skills can be enhanced by encouraging Michael to learn new words and to read more. Teaching computational skills commensurate to his grade peers should aid in improving arithmetic skills. Michael needs the supportive environment of bilingual education and ought to be evaluated bilingually, given his reliance on Spanish. Intensive instruction in all academic areas would prove beneficial at this time, given the obvious delays in all areas of academia. This is an educationally and emotionally deprived youngster who was neglected in his native country. Given the fact that emotional factors are impeding his ability to pay attention, to complete class assignments and to engage his peers socially, intensive management systems are needed in the identified academic and social skills areas. Michael is likely to do better with a lower students-to-teacher ratio and shorter exposure to teaching materials. Overall, Michael will benefit from a highly structured setting and individualized teaching methods.

SUMMARY AND RECOMMENDATIONS

Michael is a 12-year-old young man who is functioning in the borderline range of intelligence, but is of low average potential as measured by the Wechsler Intelligence Scale for Children-III. His verbal skills are borderline to low average and his nonverbal skills are low average to average. Visual-motor coordination skills are delayed as measured by the Bender test. Academic delays exist in all areas. Emotional factors are impeding learning and affecting peer relations. Michael is self-conscious about his petite body frame. Michael is clearly more proficient and dominant in Spanish. Based on the above findings, it is recommended that:

1. Michael should receive intensive instruction in all academic skills areas, in particular, math, reading and spelling. Instruction should focus on building English language skills and vocabulary/communication skills. Given his length of time in this country, his classroom placement should be a non-classified educational setting.

2. Michael should receive instruction in career awareness and career exploration.

3. Counseling aimed at building self-esteem, self-acceptance, social skills and communication skills ought to be offered.

4. Family counseling with the goal of improving parent/child communication and teaching the expression of affection ought to be provided.

5. Michael should be referred to a medical doctor to determine if there are medical difficulties that are causing the headaches and the sleep disturbances.

6. A speech/language evaluation is recommended

7. Intensive management systems, ranging from teacher-directed to student self-directed, which can lead to improvement in the identified academic and social skill areas, ought to be offered.

8. Encouraging the suspension or extension of time on demanding tasks should be done in the classroom, given his noted gains when these techniques were implemented.

9. Michael ought to be monitored closely and tested next year to see what progress he is making and whether a more/less restrictive setting would be beneficial.

Test Results – Scores

Wechsler Intelligence Scale for Children-III

Psychometric Assessment	Range	
Verbal Scale IQ	70	Borderline
Performance Scale IQ	79	Borderline
Full Scale IQ	72	Borderline

Current Verbal Scale Score		Current Nonverbal Scale Score	
Information	3	Picture Completion	7
Similarities	2	Coding	6
Arithmetic	7	Picture Arrangement	7
Vocabulary	8	Block Design	7
Comprehension	3	Object Assembly	6
Digit Span	9	Mazes	6

Wechsler Intelligence Scale for Children-III

Psychometric Potential Assessment	Range	
Verbal Scale IQ	80	Low Average
Performance Scale IQ	90	Average
Full Scale IQ	83	Low Average

Potential Scale	Score	Potential Nonverbal Scale	Score
Information	3	Picture Completion	8
Similarities	5	Coding	6
Arithmetic	9	Picture Arrangement	8
Vocabulary	10	Block Design	9
Comprehension	5	Object Assembly	11
Digit Span	9	Mazes	8

PART III

Implications for Cross-Cultural Research and Policy

Training School and University Personnel to Work with Cross-Cultural Ethnic Minority Populations

One of the major challenges facing the education field today is the training of school personnel to address the psychological needs of the increasing number of linguistic, ethnically and culturally diverse children in the school system (Barona et al., 1990; High Achieving, 1985; Reid, 1986; U.S. Department of Commerce News, 1989). Since it is virtually impossible to have an equal number of trained specialists who are themselves from the variety of culturally diverse backgrounds as our student population, it is critically important to have all school personnel be knowledgeable about and prepared to address the concerns of this diverse group of students. The goal should really be to train all school personnel to be competent, sensitive and knowledgeable of the critical factors related to issues of cultural diversity in order to best serve the culturally different. This knowledge, sensitivity and awareness ought to be built into the existing graduate training programs.

Throughout this book, many models were discussed and a bio-cultural model was proposed in working with culturally diverse children; while those are all strongly recommended, other competencies are needed as prerequisites to best utilize the model suggested herein (see Table 2).

TABLE 2   Major Multicultural Competencies for Working with Culturally Diverse Children

1. Cross-Cultural Ethical Competence
   • the treatment of culturally diverse clients by professionals who lack the specialized training and expertise is unethical.
2. Awareness of the Therapist's Own Values and Biases
   • knowledge regarding their own racial heritage and how it professionally affects the therapeutic process.
   • knowledge of how oppression and discrimination personally affects them and their work.
3. Cross-Cultural Awareness
   • acquiring awareness of the variations of different cultural groups with respect to motivational/learning styles, family roles, the impact of migration and relocation.
4. Competence in Understanding Interracial Issues
   • issues such as whether the therapist should wait for the client to introduce questions of race.
   • what are some ways that racial factors may influence the course of treatment.
5. Language Competencies
   • learn to work with bilingual clients either through the use of interpreters or by learning a second language
6. Acquiring Competency in the Ability to Work with Interpreters
   • knowledge of interpretation procedures – establishing rapport with the interpreters.
   • respecting the authority of the interpreter.
   • knowing the kinds of information that tend to get lost during the interpretation procedure.
   • recognizing the importance of securing accurate translation.
7. Cross-Cultural Assessment Competencies
   • can use assessment instruments appropriately with groups on which the tests were not standardized.
   • can articulate the limitations of the instrument with various groups.
8. Cross-Cultural Counseling Competencies
   • respect the indigenous helping beliefs and practices
   • aware of the institutional impediments that hinder the use of counseling services.
9. Cross-Cultural Issues in Conflict Resolution
   • it is necessary for the counselor to help the client to identify the ways in which conflicts affect therapy.
10. Competence in Special Education Prevention
11. Competencies in Knowing the Bilingual Education Curriculum
   • knowing what constitutes a bilingual instructional program.
12. Cross-Cultural Consultation Competencies
   • they are not adverse to seeking consultation with religious healers.
   • consult with heads of organizations that focus on providing services to individuals of different cultural groups.
13. Cross-Cultural Research Competencies
   • familiarize themselves with relevant research regarding the mental health of various ethnic and racial groups.
   • identify research that is conducted by respected professionals and viewed as credible by community members.
14. Competence in Empowering Families through Community-Based Organizations
15. Competence in Pediatric/Health Psychology
16. Competence in Parent Training

SOME COMPETENCIES NEEDED FOR CROSS-CULTURAL TRAINING

AWARENESS OF OWN CULTURAL BIASES AND VALUES

Arredondo et al. (1996) suggested that all educators and mental health workers in training should explore their fundamental significant beliefs and attitudes and the impact of those beliefs on the psychological processes and on their ability to respect others different from themselves. They should be allowed to examine their values that impede respect of others' values and beliefs. The adage "counselor know thyself" is critical in preventing ethnocentrism, a significant ingredient in effective cross-cultural counseling. Culturally competent staff ought to be trained to recognize in a teaching, assessing or counseling relationship, how and when their beliefs, attitudes and values interfere with providing the best service to their students. Likewise, training should allow them to recognize the limits of their skills and to refer the child to more appropriate resources. Training should have at its heart the ability to recognize the sources of discomfort/comfort with respect to differences in culture, ethnicity etc., and how these differences are played out in therapy. A culturally competent examiner is one who tries to avoid making negative judgments on his or her clients even if their worldview differs from that of the examiner's. In other words, they respect and appreciate their students' differences.

COMPETENCE IN UNDERSTANDING INTER-RACIAL ISSUES

"Race is an elusive, perplexing, troubling and enduring aspect of life in the United States (Carter, 1995). When a Black person introduces race into psychotherapy, it is often perceived as a form of defense or as an avoidance of a more profound issue. Given United States of America's preoccupation with race in the socio-political world, it is imperative that school personnel in training are exposed to a psychotherapeutic model that includes race (Carter, 1995). Issues such as whether the examiner should wait for the student to introduce questions of race, how should race be discussed once it has arisen, what are some ways that racial factors may influence the course of the student/personnel relationship and how can one distinguish between a racial defense and poor psychological functioning. Moreover, knowledge of racial oppression and racial discrimination should be examined in training, so that white school personnel can recognize how they benefit from institutionalized and cultural racism. Carter (1995) proposed a race inclusive model in psychotherapy. All school personnel in training should be exposed to such a model to best understand the influence of race in any relationship.

CROSS CULTURAL ISSUES IN CONFLICT RESOLUTION

The Worldview Congruence Model (Myers, 1991) discusses how interpersonal conflicts are often a result of eight worldview dimensions: psychobehavioral modality, axiology, ontology, ethos, epistemology, logic, concept of time, and concept of self. Brown & Landrum-Brown (1995) illustrated how worldview conflicts affect the student/staff/administrator triadic relationship. These conflicts may result in mistrust and resistance. Thus knowledge of one's view and that of the other party in the relationship would prove beneficial in the therapeutic and supervisory relationship. It is necessary for the administrator to help the staff and the staff to help the student to identify the ways in which these conflicts affect their relationship.

COMPETENCE IN SPECIAL EDUCATION PREVENTION

During the 1995/1996 academic school year, as we conducted several trainings throughout the State of New York, we were astounded by the sentiments expressed by many practicing psychologists and their supervisors. They repeatedly stated that even if children are not truly handicapped, they have to place them in special education in order to secure some of the services that these children need. Therefore, they diagnose these "borderline" children as learning disabled, when in fact, they do not have profiles of the typical learning disabled child. An even more disturbing issue which arose, is the sentiment that if special education no longer exists, special education teachers will become unemployed. As a result, the institution of special education is necessary, not only for the children, but for the teachers themselves. There seems to be a maintenance of this system whether it is needed or not. Of course, the fact that children in special education do not receive a high school diploma, thus hindering their chances to go on to college, does not seem to be a major concern for these professionals. To say the least, this is quite unethical and unprofessional. At this juncture, what is needed is a transitory placement for these borderline children and training for special education teachers to see themselves more as preventive workers than treatment workers. Psychologists can play a significant role in this enterprise. They can serve as consultants to school personnel in assisting special education teachers to utilize their time in working with regular education "at risk" students to prevent their placement into special education. Thus a mere paradigm shift can ensure the continued employment of special education teachers in another capacity (special education prevention specialists), and simultaneously, avoid the massive mis-placement of children in special education. Training ought to focus on the role of psychologist in expanding the role of special education teachers to the regular education setting.

ACQUIRING COMPETENCY IN THE ABILITY TO WORK WITH INTERPRETERS

In spite of every effort to secure a bilingual school personnel, at times, it is impossible to do so, given the paucity of bilingual personnel who speak "exotic" languages that are not so commonly encountered. As such, it is necessary for all school personnel to develop competencies in the interpretation procedures. Some of these skills can range from establishing rapport with the interpreters, respecting the authority of the interpreter, even if the interpreter is a teacher's aide/para-professional or a member of the Parent Teachers Association, knowing the kinds of information that tend to get lost during the interpretation procedure, understanding non-verbal communication clues, and recognizing the importance of securing accurate translation. Also evident should be knowledge of translations that are not as a result of personal evaluation by the interpreter. Moreover, "the school personnel should demonstrate the ability to plan and execute pre-service and in-service programs to prepare interpreters for work with children and to help interpreters follow ethical practices of keeping information confidential" (Figueroa et al, 1984, p. 138). It must be emphasized that unlike in a legal context, testing an individual is a more complex role for the interpreter. In the world of education and psychology non-verbal cues an be mis-interpreted if the interpreter is not familiar with the child's culture. The examiner must ensure that kinesthetic cues are not mis-interpreted by the interpreter. Figueroa et al, (1984) recommended the use of audio or video-tapes to address this situation, since a precise recording of the testing can be reviewed by the examiner after completion of the testing.

COMPETENCIES IN KNOWING THE BILINGUAL EDUCATION CURRICULUM

Knowing what constitutes a bilingual instructional program for bilingual or limited-English-proficient (LEP) children is essential in working with linguistically/culturally diverse children. There is still considerable debate as to whether an

ESL or an English immersion program is best suited to meet the needs of bilingual children (Homel, 1987). Since this debate is expected to continue for years, school personnel ought to be knowledgeable on the available programs and that some children may benefit from a certain type of program and others may benefit from another. In other words, just as there is no one single program for monolingual students, likewise, no one single program can fit all bilingual children. It is critical that this be understood by all school personnel.

COMPETENCE IN PEDIATRIC/HEALTH PSYCHOLOGY

Given the increase in the reported cases of asthma and lead poisoning in many inner-city urban schools, (Brody, 1996), it is critical that school personnel begin to explore the impact of these factors on a child's ability to learn or function effectively in the school system. This is essential in the accurate assessment of a child's handicapping condition. Ruling out any medical problems is one way of preventing misdiagnosis and misplacement.

COMPETENCE IN EMPOWERING FAMILIES THROUGH COMMUNITY BASED ORGANIZATIONS

Competent school personnel have to be able to direct their families to the community-based organizations that can support the school by utilizing their resources in working with handicapped children. After-school tutorial programs, day-care centers, free lunch programs, and free clinic care are some examples of community supports that can be used to supplement the needed services which the schools are unable to provide. Utilizing the churches, social service agencies, and other outside systems are ways of empowering the families. For example, there are after-school transportation services that can transfer children to and from therapy sessions. Tapping these community resources "is sometimes the single most important interaction in facilitating the possibility of treatment" (Boyd-Franklin, 1989, p. 156).

In addition, if certain necessary services are not available in a particular community, assisting families in forming extended family support networks should be part of the responsibility of the school personnel.

COMPETENCIES IN PARENT TRAINING

School personnel, such as mental health workers, can play a major role in educating immigrant parents about the educational and social differences in the

USA systems (Gopaul-McNicol, Thomas and Irish, 1991). They can encourage them to attend PTA meetings, explain the issues of confidentiality regarding school records, help them establish contact with community resources, and all in all, assist in the acculturation process.

All mental health workers can teach parents alternatives to corporal punishment. In summary, helping parents to understand the social and emotional adjustment difficulties their children are experiencing is of major importance in parent training.

Mental health workers also need to alert parents to the reality of special education and the need for them to question the motives of the teacher. Generally speaking, immigrant parents trust their children's teachers and allow placement in special education if the teacher recommends it. They need to be taught about the special education system, since this is a rather foreign concept to most of them. Thomas and Gopaul-McNicol (1991) discuss this in detail. In general, assisting in the acculturation process involves nine important points:

1. Education about the differences in the education and social systems, with emphasis on alternative disciplinary strategies, the meaning of educational neglect, and the importance of attending parent-teacher meetings.
2. Family empowerment, with emphasis on their legal rights.
3. Understanding the family role changes and their effect on acculturation.
4. Improving communication between parents and children.
5. Teaching parents how to build or maintain positive self-esteem in their children.
6. Coping with racism.
7. Teaching parents what support their children need at home and the importance of prioritizing their time.
8. Teaching parents how to cope with rejection from their children due to the children being embarrassed by their parents' accent.
9. Teaching immigrant parents how to endorse the concept of biculturalism, so that they do not have to live between two worlds.

The concern most often raised by parents is how to discipline children without resorting to corporal punishment. The answer involves not only teaching parents the principles of assertive discipline but, in addition, helping parents to recognize that since their children are the first generation of Americans, many of their traditional cultural values will be passed on to them. Expediting the process of "Americanization" in a radical way may leave the parents feeling stripped of cultural pride. While it is necessary for parents to understand there are laws that govern them with respect to "child abuse," they must also understand that acculturation for first-generation immigrants is a different process from acculturation for second- and third-generation immigrants. Although some of the traditional values will be passed on, inevitably, their children will not have the tremendous allegiance to their native countries as the parents do. Parents must understand that the strong cultural identity may dissipate over time, as each new generation becomes more Americanized. However, immigrant parents ought not to be expected to abandon all of their values, because this can create much anxiety and despair, leaving them vulnerable and immobilized in a sometimes hostile environment. Instead, these parents need to be taught that the essence and beauty of their culture are some of their traditional values and, to some extent, some of these values can be quite beneficial in helping children to cope. What culturally diverse children need to be taught is how to take the best from both cultures as they attempt to assimilate in their new country.

TRAINING FOR PARENTS

Via the Portage Project, Shearer and Loftin (1984) and Armour-Thomas and Gopaul-McNicol (1998) propose a guide for teacher and community leaders for how to assist parents to teach their children to enhance their children's potential at home. Structured and informal activities for the parent and the child, skilled maintenance and generalization to the community at large are offered. Sternberg (1986) offered several strategies for enhancing the memory of children, such as categorical clusters whereby an individual is taught to group things by categories instead of trying to memorize in an unordered fashion. Interactive imagery is yet another technique to aid in memorizing objects or events. If the items can not fit into a convenient category, Sternberg (1986) recommends generating the unrelated words in interactive images, such as the method of loci. Of course, remembering objects by forming acronyms from the first letter of each word can increase memory, as well.

Whitehurst, Fischel, Lonigan, Valdez-Menchaca, Arnold and Smith (1991) found that severe language problems in children can be ameliorated with a home-based intervention which uses parents as therapists. Parents were given seven standard assignments on a biweekly basis which lasted about 30 minutes for each visit. Role play and other behavioral interventions aided in the children's increasing their expressive vocabulary and this was generalized to other situations and maintained over time.

Rueda and Martinez (1992) proposed a "fiesta educativa" program, where parents play an active role through community programs to address the needs of their learning-disabled youngsters. Essentially, many Latino families worked in tandem to oversee the assessment process, the remedial services and the

overall mental health services. Educating the parents on their children's educational rights was a critical component of this program. Strom, Johnson,
Strom and Strom (1992a,b) found that schools can better serve communities
when opportunities for growth are provided to both parents and children. The
main point raised is that Latino parents can help to enhance their children's
intellectual skills by encouraging their children to ask more questions and to
experiment with problem-solving in a more independent fashion. Allowing
their children the freedom to engage in fantasy and play was also an important
technique for enhancing intelligence. In general, it was found that children's
divergent, convergent thinking, memory, and creative problem-solving were
increased by teaching these skills through a four-week (each session being two
hours in duration) parent curriculum, which was as follows:

1. The first session focused on the folly of defining giftedness via a single
criterion. Then, a more comprehensive perspective (Gardner's multiple intelligences) was presented. Before the end of this session, parents were taught how
to identify their children's other intelligences/skills/gifts.

2. The second session dealt with the kinds of activities that teachers can
use in the class to enhance critical thinking. An individualized instructional
plan for each child was shared with parents. Adequate time was allotted for
questions and answers.

3. Session three allowed parents to identify their own strengths, to evaluate
their ability to be tolerant of persistent and inopportune questions raised by
their children and their ability to be supportive of their children engaging in
conversation with adults.

4. Session four gave specific handouts to parents on how to continue
enhancing their children's intellectual potential. Guidelines for follow-up sessions were given out so parents can continue to be supportive to each other
after the group had terminated through a sort of steering committee.

We endorse programs such as the ones outlined above. However, we propose a longer training period for parents—an additional four weeks wherein
parents are taught to enhance their children's intellectual skills by exposing
them to tasks similar to the type of tasks found on IQ tests and then general-
izing these skills to the classroom.

Cultural transmission from the home to the school is essential for optimal
functioning. So if the results reveal that a child holds a particular concept in
one way, but the school ecology needs it to be reflected in another, then it is
incumbent upon the parent and the school official to train that child to master the skill in the way the school desires. For instance, when a child can put
a fan together and is unable to assemble pieces of a puzzle into a unified
whole—tasks that are conceptually quite similar—then such a child can be
directly taught through mediated learning experiences (Feuerstein, 1980; Lidz,

1991) how to transfer this knowledge from one context to another. Thus, children should be exposed to puzzles, blocks, and sequential type tasks, such as storytelling via pictures and games that have different and similar features, to help nurture abstract thinking. Parents should be encouraged to teach their children to remember in a rote manner their time tables (as is done in the British educational system) so as to develop the ability to do computations mentally. Gopaul-McNicol and Armour-Thomas (1998) offer a step-by-step practical guide to parents, teachers and community members how best to nurture and enhance the intellectual abilities of children.

Moreover, the Guidelines for Providers to the Culturally Diverse (American Psychological Association, 1993) has offered culturally relevant suggestions for practice. More community visits whereby contact is established with families, community leaders and church representatives are critical in understanding the learning styles of children and in using these systems as support to aid in the best assessment of children. In general, the research supports that children can be trained to think creatively and to enhance their intellectual potential if the appropriate intervention is put in place.

TRAINING FOR TEACHERS

Teachers' implicit theories of children's intelligence help to shape the manner they respond to them in the classroom (Murrone and Gynther, 1991). The authors found that teachers were more demanding of children with above average IQ scores as measured by standardized tests of intelligence. As such, teacher attitude and perception of intelligence tests scores need to be changed through a re-education process. Maker (1992) emphasized that "not only do standardized tests not predict success in non-academic settings, but they also are poor predictors of success in school." Maker (1992) also found that the intelligences of children can be enhanced by teaching them Tangram activities (logical mathematical reasoning) in an enrichment program.

Riley, Morocco, Gordon and Howard (1993) examined what it takes for complex ideas to become rooted in the daily instruction of teachers. The authors explored how teachers could design their curriculum to include the needs and strengths of all students. They recommended analogue experiences (writing and reading in different genres, conferencing and role-playing) to activate the children's higher cognitive abilities. They also recommended posing questions to children in a directive manner. Thus, children were always expected to develop a more elaborate type of response.

Armstrong (1994) expanded Gardner's (1993) multiple intelligences in the classroom and in so doing aided teachers in enhancing the varied skills of all children. The concern for proponents of the multiple intelligences theory is that "traditionally, schools have focused on students' analytic, mathematics and linguistic intelligence which comprise a general intelligence as measured by the IQ test" Murray (1996, p. 46). Contrary to this psychometric school of thought, the other intelligences of children are being nurtured as a form of recognizing, respecting, nurturing and enhancing the holistic intellectual potential of all children.

ATLAS (authentic teaching, learning and assessment for all students) communities is a comprehensive reform program that combines the work of four organizations—The Coalition of Essential Schools, The School Development Program, The Educational Development Center and the Development Group of Project Zero. This emphasizes all of the initiatives of these organizations—personalized learning environment, home–school collaboration, active hands-on type of learning and ongoing assessment through a curriculum-based type of approach that respond to the strengths of students.

Katz (1991) spoke of the home–school connection. She spoke of scripts that we all acquire through our experiences and through various contexts. Many children are socialized in the home to a particular script and when they enter the school setting, the script is different. So a child who was taught to be emotionally expressive in their adult–child interactions at home and who comes to the school where the interaction is emotionally cool, has to be taught a new script. This is commonly the case with many African-American children (Allen and Boykin, 1992), who were found to have more emotionally expressive experiences in their homes. The school psychologists, the teachers and the special education prevention specialists can assist such children in understanding when one script is preferred to the other. The idea should not be to inform the child that his/her script is inferior, but that in the school setting, he/she must recognize when to use which script. In other words, the child has to be taught the various scripts that he/she can use. This is analogous to a bilingual child who learns that in the classroom, he/she speaks English, but he/she can engage his/her peers socially in his/her native language. If we are going to improve learning for all children, the teachers, parents and significant others must work in a collaborative manner to bring the scripts from the home, the community and the school closer.

Adams (1989) offers thinking skills curricula, which first include ecologically valid materials such as real world experiences, followed by more abstract materials typically found on psychometric test. *The Odyssey: A Curriculum for Thinking* (Adams, 1986) focused on the foundations of reasoning, understanding language, verbal reasoning, problem-solving, decision-making and inventing thinking in a seven-part creative thinking program.

Armour-Thomas and Allen (1993) developed a cognitive training-intervention program based on Sternberg's Triarchic theory of intelligence. The purpose of the program was to help teachers understand the nature of cognitions, in this instance, (1) Sternberg's *Metacomponents, Performance Components* and *Knowledge-Acquisition components*; (2) the function of these cognitive processes in student's learning; and (3) the importance of explicitness in the use of thinking processes in three major areas of teachers' work: instructional objectives, teacher–student interactions during instruction, and assessment.

Evaluation of the program revealed certain characteristics of teachers classified as high users of process: (1) there was a consistency in their high use of process in all three stages of teaching: The objectives for their students were process-focused; (2) the interactions with students during instruction was also process-focused. The kinds of questions they asked and the quality of the feedback given to students demonstrated that not only did they model the process but they encouraged student awareness and use of these processes as well; and (3) the emphasis on process was also apparent in the way they designed their assessment procedures: variation in the format, variation in the level of complexity of the tasks, and content equivalent to what students had learned in class.

A multidisciplinary approach to enhancing the performance of children has been touted as the new model of the millennium. Haynes and Comer (1993) recommend a theme concept approach to address the needs of children. At the Yale University Child Study Center, these teams of professionals work closely with the home in a collaborative manner. This School Development Program (SDP) is at the foundation of a holistic development perspective developed by James Comer, now known as the Comer Process for Reforming Education (Comer, Haynes, Joyner and Ben-Avie, 1996). This model looks to the mental health team, the central organizing body in the school, to involve parents and teachers alike in a decision-making capacity to address the socio-cultural needs of the child. This approach is one of collaboration more than autocracy. Parents are selected by their fellow parents to represent their views on school planning. This indeed bridges the gap between the home and the school.

We endorse all of the above initiatives and, in particular, we emphasize the importance of including people from the community in effecting these change. We are increasingly mindful that the classroom is quite different from the context of the research lab, which is decontextualized and free of the ongoing activity of the typical classroom, and that while teachers are trying to include a more dynamic approach to tutelage, they are also dealing with the increase of student diversity, making teaching the most challenging vocation of our time. Enabling high levels of proficiency in cognitive competence in students will require a lot more than training in the use of process-based pedagogical strategies in planning, instruction and assessment—the major areas of the teacher's work. In addition, teacher training programs would need to provide experiences for teachers to:

> appreciate the cognitive strengths that children bring to the classroom;
> think of cognitive weaknesses as experience-specific and not as general
>   person-specific deficits;

explore ways by which children's everyday cognitions could be applied to
   school tasks;

engage teachers in self-reflective practices where they confront their
   beliefs about children whose cultural socialization may be different
   from theirs.

These experiences are likely to be rewarding to the extent that training programs forge more meaningful collaborations with the home and community so
as to more fully appreciate the other cultural niches in children's lives and
ensure that teachers are supported with extra resources in the classroom so
that they may more effectively apply information gathered from the bio-ecological assessment system.

As such, we recognize the need to share the responsibility in the schools. We
envision the psychologist as playing a prominent role in linking all of the disciplines in a multidisciplinary team approach, as outlined in the next section.

PSYCHOLOGISTS' NEW ROLE AS CONSULTANT TO PARENTS, TEACHERS, AND THE SPECIAL EDUCATION PREVENTION SPECIALISTS

At present, in the school and clinical systems, there are many professions
which function as multidisciplinary teams, in that each discipline works
almost as a separate unit and comes together primarily at Committee on
Special Education meetings, mainly to decide on placement for the child. Our
hope is that the various disciplines can begin to see the need to be more interdisciplinary than multidisciplinary (see Fig. 1).

Thus, with more interdisciplinary training, psychologists can link with
health workers so that school officials will understand how health issues
impede or enhance the child's functioning.

Likewise, psychologists can work with all school administrators to see how
their assessment findings can be used in a prescriptive manner to assist the teachers in the classroom. At this juncture, special education teachers will intervene as
special education prevention specialists. Therefore, with the help of these three
subdisciplines, children will learn to use all of their strengths to work on their
weaknesses. This should result in a reduction of special education placement.

Moreover, psychologists can liaison with the social workers and community resource people to develop a pool of resources outside of the school settings
to best empower the child and his or her family.

If the family is involved in any sort of treatment by psychotherapists/psy-
chologists/psychiatrists, etc., the psychologists can serve as a liaison and can
aid school personnel in understanding how the treatment program is enhancing or impeding the child's progress.

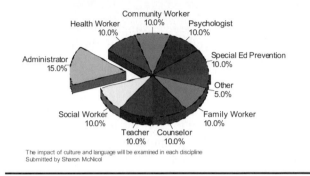

A Multi-System Interdisciplinary Model

Discipline Distribution for Successful Acculturation

Community Worker
10.0%

Health Worker
10.0%

Psychologist
10.0%

Administrator
15.0%

Special Ed Prevention
10.0%

Other
5.0%

Social Worker
10.0%

Family Worker
10.0%

Teacher   Counselor
10.0%   10.0%

The impact of culture and language will be examined in each discipline
Submitted by Sharon McNicol

Figure 1

Finally, psychologists can liaison with guidance counselors and serve in a consulting capacity, a sort of mediator between the school and vocational organizations outside of the school setting. This is to ensure that there is a connection between completion of high school and job/advanced educational opportunities.

For school psychology to survive with dignity, a multimodal, multisystems approach is needed to address the needs of people from varying ethnic/cultural backgrounds.

If such an interdisciplinary program is initiated, we envision this type of program becoming the model training program for the 21st century.

CROSS-CULTURAL COMPETENCIES AT THE UNIVERSITY LEVEL

In addition to those competencies listed above, faculty members in psychology programs need to acquire competencies in the areas listed below—consultation, supervision, research and teaching.

CROSS-CULTURAL CONSULTATION AND SUPERVISION

Cross-cultural factors that affect consultation and supervision, such as interracial therapist/client differences, language or dialectical (verbal/nonverbal) differences, social and/or occupational/economic status differences and differences due to cultural isolation (Brown and Landrum-Brown, 1995). Lefley (1986) emphasized that ongoing evaluation of counselors' multicultural development needs to be also a focus in cross-cultural training. Likewise, educational differences among the client, counselor and the supervisor, and differences in migration status and geographic origin can affect the perspectives of supervision. This is because any of these differences can affect the supervisory relationship with respect to content, process and outcome. Relatedly, these differences can result in resistance to corrective feedback because of cultural misunderstandings. This can affect the supervisory relationship to the extent that some supervisees systematically refuse to respond to the suggestions of their supervisors in order to maintain the cultural relevance of their therapeutic approaches.

Brown and Landrum-Brown (1995) outlined and critiqued several supervision theories that consider the relevant cross-cultural dimensions that are likely to influence the supervisory process. What is still desperately needed is an expansion of these supervisory models to embody the intercultural dynamic interaction.

Family consultation is in dire need of addressing since the concept of family has changed immensely over the past 15 years. Thus, the nuclear family with two parents and two children no longer exists. Many cultures emphasize the extended family as a strong financial and emotional support system (Halsell Miranda, 1993). In general, psychologists should be able to assist both teachers and parents in planning, implementing and following-up on the child's individual educational program.

CROSS-CULTURAL TEACHING—A PROPOSED MULTICULTURAL CURRICULUM

Bernal and Padilla (1982) called for a multicultural training philosophy. The competencies described above should be infused into the existing graduate program, with each student receiving a one-year internship in a multiethnic/multicultural/multilinguistic school district. In addition, the curriculum should take on a more interdisciplinary approach, utilizing the contributions from related fields such as social work, psychiatry, and anthropology. Intradiscipline by way of exposure to cross-cultural issues in clinical, counseling, social, developmental and educational psychology can be quite beneficial in cross-cultural training. Moreover, focusing on areas such as psycholinguistics, bilingual/multicultural education, cross-cultural theory, and cross-cultural counseling are all necessary requisites in developing cross-cultural competence. Ethical/legal issues in multicultural assessment, treatment, consultation, supervision, research, etc. should be infused in each course, not offered only as a separate course. Ridley (1985) suggested that every effort should be made to ferret out the principles that are universal in nature, so that a basis for determining where cultural variability begins and cultural generalization ends would be established. Exposure to various cultural groups should afford students the opportunity to be part of a viable programmatic experience.

Rogers et al. (1992) found that 60% of the doctoral and non-doctoral programs they surveyed offered merely one course specifically devoted to multicultural issues and 63% of those programs surveyed offered two to five courses. Seventy-five percent of the programs made at least one multicultural course a requirement. Rogers et al. (1992) also found that 27% of the programs they surveyed spent less than 5% of their time on courses related to minority issues. Forty percent did not spend any time at all on courses addressing a multicultural content, and most of the programs (94%) did not require exposure to a foreign language course. As such, the need to develop a specific multicultural curriculum is crucial.

IMPLEMENTATION OF THE CURRICULUM

To accomplish this innovative multicultural training program, a step-by-step guideline is outlined below.

1. A written academic policy emphasizing a clear statement of purpose and commitment to cultural diversity, as well as the consequences to the program if these policies are violated. Included in this statement must be definite quantifiable, tangible program objectives that must be achieved within a particular time frame.

2. Inclusion of cultural and ethnic content should be infused in each course, not taught as a single course only. Thus, psychological assessment should be first taught, whereby students are exposed to adherence to standardized procedures, and then they should be taught how to step away from standardized testing. Likewise, treatment should allow for cultural consideration throughout the therapeutic courses.

3. There should be a more aggressive recruitment of faculty members and students of various cultural backgrounds. Working with an ethnically diverse student and faculty body adds enrichment to the program since one can view issues from various perspectives.

4. Faculty members should be encouraged to update their cross-cultural expertise by attending continuation education courses, seminars, etc. The university should give a reduction in their teaching load for one year to allow for this cross-cultural training.

5. A consultant or a full-time faculty member with cross-cultural expertise should be available to consult with all faculty members to assist them in redesigning their curriculum to reflect a diverse cultural content.

6. Funds should be set aside for a few research students to be assigned strictly for this cross-cultural thrust—building a cross-cultural resource file, assisting in student and faculty recruitment, linking with community people to recruit more ethnic minority practicum supervisors, coordinating experts of different cultural backgrounds to speak at colloquia, etc.

7. Both a faculty member and several students should be allotted to represent ethnic students' concerns.

8. Form linkages with other departments within the university structure to identify existing cross-cultural courses and experts in the cross-cultural studies.

9. Faculty members should be encouraged to attend international conferences not only in European countries, but in developing countries as well.

10. For the first two years, an ongoing review of the program to ensure that the goals are being met should be done on a monthly basis at regular staff meetings. After two years of smooth functioning, it should be done on a quarterly basis, and after five years, an annual basis should suffice. Every faculty member should be required to sit in on these meetings.

11. Without all of the above in place and without financial support to fund all of these innovative efforts, failure is most likely to occur. Since the ultimate goal of innovation should be institutionalization, then hard-line financial endowments are needed (Ridley, 1985).

Johnson (1982, 1987, 1990) developed a two-part course that included theory, current research and a laboratory experiential section. Practica in all areas of their training should be available to ensure that all students receive hands-on training in working with culturally/linguistically different children. Rogers et al. (1992) found that 69% of program directors estimated that students were exposed to minority clients less than a quarter percent of their time during their practicum and internship experiences. Even more concerning, they found that almost one-third of the programs surveyed reported that students spent 0–5% of their experiential training time with minority clients. This suggests that a large percentage of "school psychology students have limited or no direct exposure to culturally diverse clients during field training" (p. 607). Mio (1989), in his multicultural counseling course, allowed students to interact with a person from a different culture on a regular basis over the course of the semester. It was found that these students who were matched with immigrant students were rated as more culturally sensitive at the end of the semester. Clearly, the experiential component helps promote cultural awareness and knowledge of another culture.

A multicultural curriculum should be multifaceted, consisting of a combination of assessment, review of the ethnic literature, personal involvement and the development of a small classroom group project (Parker et al., 1986). This approach utilizes the cognitive, affective and behavioral domains. The students should first be assessed on their knowledge, attitudes and perceptions of cross-cultural experiences, as well as on their comfort level in interacting with others from different ethnic/racial groups. This assessment process serves as a guide to the professor for future training. Part two of the course involves the readings and discussions about the racial/ethnic literature. Part three is very action-oriented, in that it involves behavioral activities geared to helping students increase cultural knowledge, sensitivity and effectiveness. Students initially observe from a distance videotapes, etc., and gradually move to participate directly. In the final stage, the students are expected to work on a small group activity in class. Such a project allows the students to become aware of their own stereotypical values about other racial/ethnic groups.

Cross-cultural training should also focus on the influence of race in racial identity development (Carter, 1995). Carter makes recommendations for white professors who teach multicultural students and cross-cultural issues, as well as minority professors who teach cross-cultural issues to a white student population.

In conclusion, in order to prevent the marginalization of the education and psychology professions, there is a dire need to make some serious changes to address the growing change in the population demographics, in particular in the metropolitan areas. A true commitment to cross-cultural training requires at minimum the implementation of all of the above. If a cross-cultural training program has only the bare skeleton of a commitment, then this creates no more than false generosity (Freire, 1970), dishonesty and continued disrespect. The goal should be to produce competent school personnel capable of working with children from any linguistic, cultural or ethnic background.

CHAPTER 13

Implications for Cross-Cultural Research in Assessment

A common theme throughout this book is that standardized assessment is inappropriate for children from culturally and linguistically diverse backgrounds. The problem is both conceptual and methodological. While we acknowledge that, in part, psychological functioning is rooted in biology, how these biological potentials unfold and the trajectory of their development is under the control of culture. The inextricable linking of biology and culture makes constructs like intelligence, language, and personality bio-cultural phenomena and, therefore, should be assessed with procedures consistent with this conceptualization. Although there are research findings that are supportive of the cultural dependency of cognition, language, and personality, a number of methodological challenges remain. A discussion of some of these issues follows.

UNPACKAGE CULTURAL ATTRIBUTES WITHIN SOCIAL GROUPS

One of the problems of standardized assessment is that assessment developers often use concepts (e.g., race, ethnicity, and socioeconomic status) as if they were interchangeable with culture. More than twenty years ago, Whiting (1976) referred to these concepts as packaged variables that serve as labels that represent psychologically salient experiences for individuals and groups who identify with them. More recently, Gauvain (1995) clarified the nature of the dilemma that the cultural labels pose for researchers.

> It is difficult to fit culture into a methodology that divides reality into independent and dependent variables. Culture is clearly inappropriate as a dependent variable, but it is equally problematic to consider it an independent variable ... culture cannot be randomly assigned to research participants and, therefore, the basic assumption of independence is violated (pg. 26).

There are two methodological difficulties associated with the unpackaging of psychological processes associated with culture that would need to be empirically investigated. The first has to do with the differential experiencing of culture as a function of its association with other dimensions of human diversity. In other words, the relationship between culture and class, culture and ethnicity, and culture and language needs to be better understood in ways that allow for the observation of meaningful differences within and among cultural groups. Next, the dimensions of culture that have psychological implications need to be operationally defined at a level of detail sufficient to permit measurement. In this way, culturally defined roles, beliefs, and attitudes may be subjected to comparative analysis within and among cultural groups.

ENSURE CULTURAL EQUIVALENCE IN ASSESSMENT PROCEDURES

The second problematic assumption underlying standardized tests is that comparisons between social groups can be made since items are written in ways that do not favor any particular experience. Consequently, any observed differences are reflective of factors intrinsic to the individual. But as we have argued throughout this book, dimensions of human development (e.g., intellectual, personality, and language) unfold within a cultural niche and, therefore, behavior at any point in time is a product of cultural socialization. If we must compare performance between members whose cultural socialization differs, then every effort must be made to ensure cultural equivalence in assessment measures used to appraise the construct of interest. Lonner (1981) identified four types of equivalence that should be addressed when making comparisons between distinctive cultural groups:

> functional equivalence: whether the psychological construct operates in the same manner for cultural groups and test scores have the same meaning for different cultural groups

linguistic equivalence: the extent to which language used in tests have the
   same meaning for different cultural groups
conceptual equivalence: the extent to which task attributes have the same
   meaning for different cultural groups
psychometric equivalence: whether tests measure psychological characteristics at the same levels in different cultural groups

Given the relative inattention to these issues in standardized tests, they are
worthwhile areas for research for assessment developers.

SEEK A CLEARER UNDERSTANDING
OF CULTURAL NICHES

Yet another faulty assumption of standardized tests is that observed differences in behavior in a testing context are not necessarily indicative of differences intrinsic to the individual or group. Although we have come to appreciate the situatedness of human functioning, we are still relatively uninformed
about the mechanisms by which the various subsystems with a cultural niche
(value system, language system, symbol system) function to account for differential development and behavior. More fine-grained ethnographic research
is needed to determine how these subsystems create regularities in the environment in ways that enable meaningful learning. Just as important, we need
to identify the conditions and interactions that contribute to irregularities in
ways that impede learning. Only then should comparative judgment be made
regarding observations of within- and between-group differences for any
behavior of interest.

REEXAMINE EPISTEMOLOGICAL ASSUMPTIONS

Perhaps the most serious problem of standardized assessment may have less to
do with identifying cultural attributes, testing contexts, or cultural equivalences than with the epistemological assumptions underlying such procedures.
Epistemologies or theories of knowledge describe assumptions about the
nature of our world and our experiences of it. In countries where a dominant
culture coexists with subordinate cultures, members of the dominant and sub-
ordinated cultures have different epistemologies (Collins, 1991; Gordon et al.,
1990; Scheurich and Young, 1997). As a function of their divergent structural
positions, sociopolitical histories and experiences (Stanfield, 1985), these epistemological assumptions are not value-free nor inconsequential. As Gordon et
al. (1990, p.15) have argued, the tendency of the dominant group is to

make one's own community the center of the universe and the conceptual frame
that constrains all thought. This communicentricity has sometimes resulted in
knowledge production and utilization that has negative consequences for the life
experiences of groups who have been inappropriately represented in the enterprise.

The relative neglect of the experiences of children socialized beyond the pale
of the dominant culture of the U.S. in standardized assessment processes suggests that assessment developers and users empirically reexamine the epistemological assumptions of their practices.

OTHER SUGGESTIONS FOR FUTURE RESEARCH

Personality

1. Examine the folk beliefs in assessing the personality of clients from culturally diverse backgrounds, especially as applies to paranoid schizophrenia.

Language

1. English as a second dialect versus English as a second language ought to
be examined in light of the controversy over Ebonics and Creole speakers versus bilingual speakers.

2. The notion that different representational language systems may differentially influence language acquisition suggests a need for comparative
research regarding children's exposure to different language structures.

Intelligence

1. The responsiveness of cognitive potentials to environmental stimulation
suggests a need for more systematic studies regarding the trainability of intellectual skills.

2. The finding that children demonstrate intelligences other than those
assessed on IQ tests suggests the need for research regarding the kinds of experiences likely to nurture spatial, musical and bodily-kinesthetic intellectual
competencies.

Academic Achievement

1. The finding that differential prior educational experiences influence academic functioning suggests the need for investigating the effects of equivalent
exposure to the same instructional content for different cultural groups.

2. The finding that when classroom practices are compatible with the practices of the natal culture children learn well, suggests the need for more pre-

cise definition of those cultural features and for studying variations in classroom practice as a function of these compatible cultural practices.

Vocation

To date, very little has been done in the area of vocational assessment of cross-ethnic and cross-cultural populations. Evidently, like all standardized tests, items on vocational tests are lacking in cultural equivalencies. Research to determine the cultural differences in responding to test questions is needed. Moreover, the disproportionate number of clients from culturally diverse backgrounds in blue-collar career settings suggests the need to reexamine the assumptions of these measures for this population of clients.

CONCLUSION

It is inconceivable that an assessment measure could be reliable and valid if its conceptual foundation is faulty. We think, as many other researchers do, that standardized tests rest on a flawed understanding of human development and behavior as pertains to intelligence, language, academic achievement and personality. The assessment practice of making comparative judgments between cultural distinct groups is premature since insufficient research attention has been given to the impact of cultural differences on the development and expression of behavior in these realms. More systematic research about these constructs is needed, particularly for children socialized beyond the pale of U.S. mainstream culture.

CHAPTER 14

Policy Implications in Cross-Cultural Assessment

At present, in the school and clinical systems, there are many disciplines which function as multidisciplinary teams. Our concern is that each discipline work almost as a separate unit, and that they come together primarily at Committee on Special Education meetings, mainly to decide on placement for the child.

Our hope is that the various disciplines can begin to see the need to be more interdisciplinary than multidisciplinary (see Fig. 1). With more interdisciplinary training, administrators can link with health workers so that school officials will understand how these factors are impeding or enhancing the child's functioning. For the mental health field to survive with respect, a multimodal, multisystems approach is needed to address the needs of people from diverse ethnic/cultural backgrounds.

ISSUES IN POLICY DEVELOPMENT

Dunn (1978) defines policy as the outcome of decision-making processes set in motion to respond to existing challenges. In educational policy-making, an individual or group of individuals who hold similar beliefs and have similar needs want something from government or other agencies and builds a coalition of influence to obtain it (Bransford and Baca, 1989). They strategize and develop tactics intended to provoke decision-makers and those in power to pass laws and issue executive and judicial orders to address their needs and concerns (Bransford and Baca, 1989). The most critical issues impacting policy development are financing, states' rights issues or local control, planning and implementation, training needs, and effectiveness of instructional strategies and educational programs (Bransford and Baca, 1989).

Today, in light of the dwindling financial resources available to local school districts to develop effective programs aimed at addressing the educational needs of all children, for culturally and linguistically diverse students, the monies allocated are even smaller. Cutbacks in funding from the federal government have been met with a certain hesitancy by local educational agencies to assume the cost because they do not have the resources. When the federal government shifts the responsibility of education to the states and local agencies, culturally and linguistically diverse student population are generally the first to feel the reduction in educational services. School districts in high poverty areas are usually the ones with the greatest needs and the least financial resources to address those needs, while more affluent districts do not have the number of culturally and linguistically diverse populations that would motivate them to create programs for this population. In either case, programs designed to answer the educational needs of culturally and linguistically diverse students are few.

There is an ongoing debate between the federal government and state agencies regarding the responsibility of educating the children of this nation. One of the main arguments used by the states' rights advocates is that educating the children of America has long been the recognized constitutional responsibility of the states and local school districts (Thompson and Hixson, 1984). They maintain that the Department of Education issues specific guidelines and statutes that have usurped the power of the states and local school boards to determine educational strategies and curriculum policies. Bransford and Baca (1989) argued that the lack of coordination between federal and state agencies in planning, implementation, and evaluation of programs has led to weak guidelines for program monitoring, wasted human and material resources and a failure to address students' individual educational needs.

Cummins (1984) warned that changes in beliefs and attitudes among educational practitioners can result only from the actual process of carrying out different approaches, where the evidence of their appropriateness is allowed to speak for itself. Moreover, at the level of policy-making, parents' involvement in the community, school, and grassroots political organizations would place political pressures on policy-makers to enact legislative acts whose goal is to strengthen and build the educational options of culturally and linguistically diverse students so that the students can succeed to their fullest potential.

IMPLICATION FOR POLICY-MAKERS

Throughout this book, the authors have discussed a number of strategies in the areas of assessment, and educational interventions to improve the educational performance of culturally diverse students. This chapter briefly recapitulates the approaches endorsed in light of their implications for culturally diverse students, their teachers, other school personnel and policy-makers. The research had delineated pedagogical and assessment strategies that may provide a guide for the development of future educational policies, which would, in turn, lay a foundation for educational practices.

The responsibility to adequately educate all children falls upon the shoulders of the federal government, local school districts, communities, teachers, and parents. However, it is clear that children who live in the less affluent school districts of the nation attend schools that are overcrowded with limited educational resources, such as outdated textbooks, insufficient number of books per student, high student-to-teacher ratios in remedial and bilingual programs, inadequate level of services (e.g., remedial reading instruction in a large group once a week), inadequately administered programs, and dilapidated school buildings. As Cummins (1984) argues, policy-makers must realize that the causes of culturally diverse students are both varied and complex. However, while no one factor can be identified as the sole culprit, research has identified a number of factors that operate together in such a way that predictions can be made (Cummins, 1984); consequently, policy-makers can create and fund programs that would prevent the failure of culturally diverse students. Several factors have been identified as contributors to the school failure of these students:

LACK OF PARENT AND COMMUNITY INVOLVEMENT

Parent and community involvement in school programs generates support for programs aiming at addressing the needs of these students, not only at the local level but also in terms of political pressure to fund these programs. Additionally, parent involvement, such as school staff working with parents to establish an atmosphere in the home that is conducive to learning, is essential to children's success in school. Educators who can establish a relationship of trust and mutual respect with parents of culturally and linguistically diverse students will be able to involve parents in the process of building literacy skills in their children (Cummins, 1984). Teachers and parents must be partners in the education of children. Therefore, teachers must be knowledgeable about the cultural beliefs and practices of parents and community. They must know how to accommodate the cultural diversity that may exist and be able to communicate with parents in their native language or with the use of an interpreter. Policy-makers must encourage and provide the financial allocation so the local school districts may develop parent involvement programs.

When linguistically and culturally diverse students continue to experience difficulty in achievement, most teachers' first step is to refer that student to special education. Although, IDEA requests that the referring party document prereferral interventions, teachers often consider ESL and bilingual education as a prereferral intervention. Gartner (1986) emphasized this point and submits that the present system has no structured procedure in place to determine the validity of a referral and that the system provides very little incentive for preventing special education placement. As a matter of fact, teachers are encouraged by school administrators to refer low-achieving students to special education, so that their scores on statewide or districtwide competency exams are not added to their school's overall performance. The unreal pressure that school administrators feel to meet minimal competency standards set up by the state promotes a pressured, competitive classroom atmosphere that maximizes the risk of academic failure for students with potential academic difficulties (Cummins, 1984). It encourages teachers to "teach to the test" and teachers have very little time to inclination to modify instruction or to accommodate the educational needs of at-risk students.

Gardner (1989) argues that most special education students could be better served in a fully mainstreamed program if they were provided with greater attention to individual needs, adaptation of learning environments to accommodate diversity, train and support school personnel to respond to student diversity, and fund efforts aimed at prevention. In many instances, teachers (for lack of guidance as to how to provide prereferral services and modify instruction) wait until students who exhibit minor gaps in achievement fall substantially below grade level to make a referral for special education. Other times, the student is referred a number of times until he or she qualifies (based on state criteria as to what constitutes a learning impairment) for special education services. During the "waiting" period, the struggling student is provided with little or no educational service to remediate the problem. These practices should be considered educational malpractice and teachers and administrators should be accountable.

While the current amendment to IDEA (U.S. Department of Education, 1995) recognizes the need to fund prevention programs and include special education students in all assessments, most school districts have not been responsive in developing programs to address culturally and linguistically diverse students' needs. Federal and state funding formulas must help promote good practices in education and this include special education prevention programs (U.S. Department of Education, 1995).

TRADITIONAL PEDAGOGICAL STRATEGIES

If cooperative learning approaches have been found to be effective with culturally and linguistically diverse students who share a cultural worldview that embraces cooperative and noncompetitive values and lifestyles, then why is it that most teachers who work with this student population are not implementing these strategies in their classrooms? Why is it that if research supports the use of context in teaching language arts, most teachers still rely on a decontextualized teaching strategy to impart their lessons? Moreover, the research is rather clear in terms of the benefit of using culturally relevant instructional material and the use of context in learning new information; yet most culturally and linguistically diverse students are given instructional materials that are culturally alien. Consequently, children have difficulty connecting emotionally, cognitively, socially, and linguistically with the information, and this interferes with learning. Undoubtedly, many of the culturally and linguistically diverse students identified as "learning disabled" exhibit learning difficulties that are pedagogically induced (Cummins, 1984).

Policy-makers should recognize the need for multicultural instructional materials, through executive orders, rules and regulations, or even public speeches or endorsements. This would, in turn, put pressure on the publishers of textbooks and instructional material to develop multicultural educational materials that recognize the cultural heritage of students and on local school districts to purchase these materials. Policy-makers should take responsibility for promoting and transmitting instructional models that have shown positive results with culturally and linguistically diverse students.

EXIT CRITERIA FOR ESL PROGRAMS

Limited English-proficient students are exited from ESL programs based on their score on a language proficiency test. Limited English-proficient students are usually mainstreamed into a full English curriculum after two to three years in a ESL program. Students who continue to score low on their language proficiency test are typically referred to Special Education. Although research has found that when children have been exited from these programs, they usually have only achieved BICS (i.e., basic interpersonal communication skills) and not CALP (i.e., cognitive academic language proficiency), educational policy has not changed to recognize this fact. It is not uncommon for LEP students who have been exited from ESL to continue to have learning problems because they have not achieved the type of cognitive language proficiency necessary for full comprehension and fast processing of academic facts in English. It is an accepted notion that it takes between 5 and 7 years for LEP students to approach grade-level performance in English verbal academic skills (Cummins, 1984). However, children are still expected to function up to par with their monolingual English peers. Limited English proficient students experience most of their learning difficulties in content area courses, such as social studies and science, where classes are heavily language-based and use unfamiliar vocabulary. Policy-makers must develop an extension to ESL programs (e.g., a transitional program) and interventions where children are provided with academic and linguistic support to facilitate the development of CALP.

One such intervention is the Sheltered English Program, and its approach appears effective for teaching academic courses to LEP (Watson et al., 1989). In this program, teachers incorporate second language acquisition principles with traditional teaching strategies to increase the comprehensibility of the lesson for students (Krashen, 1982). Teachers make many adjustments, for example, they preteach two vocabularies: the words necessary to understand the content of the lesson and the words used to explain the lesson (Watson et al., 1989). Teachers use the same lesson format in order to provide a structure for learning, which reduces the time necessary for the students to decipher how the teacher is presenting new material (Watson et al., 1989). Manipulative and visual techniques are used to illustrate the concepts. Cooperative learning techniques are utilized, and they provide the interactive aspect that brings lessons to life and enhances learning. Additionally, students are instructed on learning strategies or study skills: note taking, listening skills, and outlining (Watson et al., 1989). Research on Sheltered English Programs have shown positive results (Watson et al., 1989).

INADEQUATE EDUCATIONAL SUPPORT

Limited English-proficient students are provided with either ESL or bilingual education, and in some cases, they might be offered remedial reading in addition to ESL or bilingual education. Once children are exited from ESL or bilingual education, the only other support program available is remedial reading. However, strategies used in remedial reading are usually not effective since they do not individualize instruction or target entry-level skills.

Policy-makers should introduce educational legislative acts that endorse more individualized instruction in remedial reading or Chapter one services.

Research has found that the most effective remedial programs are those that provide tutorial or one-to-one instruction and where the students' skills are assessed and re-assessed frequently (e.g., every 8 to 10 weeks) to readjust instructional goals and strategies.

LACK OF APPROPRIATE EDUCATIONAL PLANNING FOR OVERAGE STUDENTS

Unfortunately, there is an increasing number of immigrant students who arrive in the United States with little to no educational background. These children present an even greater challenge to the public schools when they are overage (e.g., a seventeen-year-old 10th-grader). These students are quickly frustrated by the educational system and they drop out of school. Many times, the first course of action is to simply refer these children to special education in order to provide them individualized or small group instruction and remediation. However, most of these students are not disabled children in need of special education services. The lack of appropriate programming to address their needs seems to be the crux of the problem.

Individualized or small group instruction appears to be the most effective type of educational intervention for overage students. In developing a program for these students, several components are essential: home/school connection to develop trust and a bond with the family; study strategies must be taught; building self-esteem by including the student in the planning and accessing their wishes and desires for their future; vocational and career planning; work-study programs; cooperative learning strategies, to reduce isolation and allow the student to discuss his or her life experience; use mutlicultural instructional materials; build basic literacy skills; frequent assessment to tailor instruction to students' needs; develop language skills; and use multiple strategies to illustrate and demonstrate concepts.

LACK OF COMPREHENSIVE ASSESSMENT MODELS

Over the years, professional organizations such as the American Psychological Association and the National Council of Measurement in Education have reflected concerns regarding discriminatory practices in intelligence testing through their *Bylaws, Ethical Principles,* and *Standards.* However, these noble sentiments seem to have had minimal impact on the construction of standardized tests or the practice of psychology. As indicated in Chapter 3, interpretation and use of test results have been particularly inimical to ethnic and linguistic children, particularly those from low-income backgrounds. It is as if test developers and practitioners have been oblivious to the theoretical and empirical research regarding the situatedness of cognition over the last two decades and to the influence of linguistic and cultural diversity in intelligent behavior. But, even more disheartening, they seem unaware of the devastating consequences of their judgments, which place large numbers of children on educational paths that are neither enabling nor worth wanting. Indeed, the literature is replete with inequitable schooling of children placed in low-track classes or in unwarranted special educational programs (Kozol, 1991; Lipsky and Gartner, 1996; Oakes, 1990). Perhaps a list of principles and standards, no matter how well intentioned, is insufficient insurance against discriminatory practice in standardized testing. What is needed, in our judgment, is greater democratic reciprocity in discussions among practitioners, test developers, and client representatives in the development of principles and standards-setting with respect to assessment practices. Equally important is the need for enforceable principles that are truly reflective of our commitment to equity and cultural pluralism. Though not exhaustive, we submit the following questions for consideration:

> Are the principles and standards essentially and sufficiently accommodating of multiple cultural perspectives?
>
> Are the principles and standards supportive of multiple expressions of intelligent behavior?
>
> Are the principles and standards supportive of the assessment of cognitive potential?
>
> Are the principles and standards supportive of evidence of intelligence and personality beyond the standardized testing context?
>
> Do the principles and standards provide clear implications for desirable competencies among practitioners, both psychologists in training and practicing psychologists/clinicians?
>
> Are there mechanisms for the incorporation of these competencies in accreditation criteria?

Legislative acts and statutes should specify and define what is involved in non-biased or nondiscriminatory assessment. For example, legislative statutes must delineate that as part of a nondiscriminatory assessment, school psychologists and educational educators must use testing strategies that modify standard testing procedures when necessary to accommodate bilingual and bicultural issues. Extensive background information should be gathered. This includes data about acculturation, immigration experiences, community lifestyle, religious affiliations and belief, academic background or school history, medical history, parents' educational background and ideas about education, social experiences in the country of origin and language exposure.

Poor Training of Future Educational Practitioners at the University and College Levels

Very few university programs that train teachers, school psychologists, speech and language pathologists, etc. do not have a true commitment to preparing teachers that are ready to work with culturally and linguistically diverse populations. These new educational practitioners do not understand the special issues that impact on this population: second language acquisition, acculturation process, and historical events. More importantly, teachers' lack of understanding leads them to view culturally and linguistically diverse students as deficient instead of being able to appreciate their differences and use it to enrich their learning. The failure to see the potential of these children results in the underestimation of their cognitive abilities, which limits their educational options.

Teachers, school administrators, and psychologists and other educational practitioners in training are only required to take one course in multicultural issues as part of their preparation. The implication here is that the understanding of multicultural issues is not important enough to warrant more required courses or a multicultural component to every course in their core curriculum.

Policy-makers must allocate funding to universities and colleges to encourage multicultural and bilingual training programs that would prepare future educational practitioners to work with culturally and linguistically diverse students and families. Teachers, school psychologists, speech and language pathologists and other educational practitioners should be certified to work with culturally and linguistically diverse students. Therefore, local school districts should be encouraged to provide inservice or require further training of their school personnel by offering salary incentives or tuition reimbursement for additional training in this area and to obtain certification to work with this population.

Accountability

Local school districts and policy-makers must be accountable and responsible for providing an appropriate education to culturally and linguistically diverse students. This means that the local school district should be able to modify its already existing resources to accommodate the educational needs of these students. For example, current remedial reading or Chapter 1 services can be modified to accommodate culturally and linguistically diverse students by using instructional techniques that have shown positive results with this population. Policy-makers can provide sufficient flexibility in their funding criteria that would allow local school districts to also service the need of culturally and linguistically diverse students. According to Slavin (1988), in light of the increasing number of student failures, schools often blame parents, society, television, or the students themselves. Although societal factors do make educating children a more difficult task, schools still hold the greater responsibility in ensuring that children attending their institutions succeed.

Slavin (1988) emphasized several factors where schools have definite control:

1. *Focus on prevention:* from the onset, schools should see to it that every child learns to read by providing appropriate instruction (e.g., varied and culturally sensitive instructional strategies, emphasizing language development). Structured preschool and kindergarten programs provide the foundation children need when they are beginning to read in the first grade; moreover, it is in the first grade that intensive remedial programs should begin (Slavin 1988).

2. *Focus on classroom change:* The gains made by preschool and kindergarten educational experience should be followed with appropriate instruction in the classrooms. Again, the use of culturally sensitive instructional material and the use of varied manipulatives and visual techniques to illustrate educational concepts, as well as the development of language skills.

3. *Focus on the appropriate use of remedial programs:* the implementation of a remedial program after the student has fallen two to three grade levels behind usually does not make a significant impact on reducing the gap. These programs should be used when they are most effective, which is when the child begins to show a lag in the mastery of basic academic skills. Intensive remediation should be offered then.

Policy-makers and local school districts should take a closer look at the manner in which programs are used and implemented in the schools so that they address the educational needs of all students. Policy-makers should be accountable for relying heavily on quantitative indices (e.g., statewide and districtwide standardized competency tests) to determine minimal competency because, in so doing, they have ignored the quality of instruction in the classroom (Cummins, 1984), and this has contributed to the high rate of failure of culturally and linguistically diverse students in school. Most importantly, although research in second language acquisition has supported the view that students' English and academic skills developed more rapidly and solidly in strong bilingual programs, policy-makers have ignored the merits of this approach because bilingual classes are still a source of much controversy in the United States. Unfortunately, the controversy over bilingual education is not about the effectiveness of this program and instructional approach, instead, it is rooted in nationalistic concerns and even prejudice.

REFERENCES

Adams, M. J. (1989). Thinking skills curricula: Their promise and progress. *Educational Psychologist, 24(1)*, 25–75.

Allen, B. A., & Boykin, A. W. (1992). Children and the educational process: Alienating cultural discontinuity through prescriptive pedagogy. *School Psychology Review, 21(4)*, 586–596.

Allington, R. L. (1990). Teacher interruption behaviors during primary-grade oral reading. *Journal of Educational Psychology, 72*, 371–374

Alva, S. (1993). Differential patterns of achievement among Asian-American adolescents. *Journal of Youth and Adolescence, Vol. 22(4)*, 407–423.

Ambursley, F., & Cohen, R. (1983). *Crises in the Caribbean*. New York: Monthly Review Press.

American Psychiatric Association (1987). *Diagnostic and statistical manual of mental disorders* (3rd ed. revised). Washington, DC: Author.

American Psychological Association. (1981). Ethical principles of psychologists. *American Psychologist, 36*, 633–681.

American Psychological Association. (1993). Guidelines for providers of psychological services to ethnic, linguistic and culturally diverse populations. *American Psychologist, 48*, 45–48.

Anderson, W., & Grant, R. (1987). *The new newcomers*. Toronto: Canadian Scholars Press.

Aponte, H. (1976). The family-school interview: An ecostructural approach. *Family Process, 15(3)*, 303–311.

Aponte, H., & Van Deusen, J. (1981). Structural family therapy. In A. Gurman & D. Kniskern (eds.), *Handbook of family therapy*. New York: Brunner/Mazer.

Armour-Thomas, E. (1992a). Assessment in the service of thinking and learning for low achieving students. *High School Journal* (in press).

Armour-Thomas, E. (1992b). Intellectual assessment of children from culturally diverse backgrounds. *School Psychology Review, 21(4)*, 552–565.

Armour-Thomas, E., & Allen, B. (1993). The feasibility of an information-processing methodology for the assessment of vocabulary competence. *Journal of Instructional Psychology, 20(4)*, 306–313.

Armour-Thomas, E., & Gopaul-McNicol, S. (1997a). A bio-ecological approach to intellectual assessment. *Cultural Diversity and Mental Health, Vol. 3. No. 2*, 25–39.

Armour-Thomas, E., & Gopaul-McNicol, S. (1997b). Examining the correlates of learning disability: A bio-ecological approach. *Journal of Social Distress and the Homeless, VOl. 6. No. 2*. 140–165.

Armour-Thomas, E., & Gopaul-McNicol, S. (1998). *Assessing intelligence: Applying a bio-cultural model*. Thousand Oaks, CA: Sage Publications.

175

Armstrong, T. (1994). *Multiple intelligences in the classroom.* Alexandria, VA: Association for Supervision and Curriculum Development.

Arredondo, P., Toporek, R., Pack Brown, S., Jones, J., Locke, D., Sanchez, J., & Stadler, H. (1996). Operationalization of the multicultural counseling competencies. *Journal of Multicultural Counseling and Development, 24(1),* 42–78.

Arredondo-Down, P. (1981). Personal loss and grief as a result of migration. *The Personnel and Guidance Journal, 58,* 376–378.

Asante, M. K. (1987). *The afrocentric idea.* Philadelphia: Temple University Press.

Asby, D. (1975). Empathy: Let's get the hell on with it. *The Counseling Psychologist, 5(2),* 10–15.

Au, K. (1980). Participation structures in a reading lesson with Hawaiian children. *Anthropology and Education Quarterly, 11,* 91–115.

Au, K. H. (1993). *Literacy instruction in multicultural settings.* Forth Worth, TX: Harcourt Brace Jovanovich.

Auerswald, E. (1968). Interdisciplinary versus ecological approach. *Family Process, 7,* 204.

Avolio, B., & Waldman, D. (1994). Variations in cognitive, perceptual and psychomotor abilities across the working life span: Examining the effects of race, sex, experience, education and occupational type. *Psychology and Aging, Vol. 9(3),* 430–442.

Bache, R. M. (1895). Reaction time with reference to race. *Psychological Review, 11,* 474–486.

Backler, A., & Eakin, S. (1993). *Every child can succeed: Readings for school improvement.* Bloomington, IN: Agency for Instructional Technology.

Baker, E. L. (1991). Developing comprehensive assessments of higher order thinking. In G. Kulm, (Ed.), *Assessing higher order thinking in mathematics.* Washington, DC: American Association for the Advancement of Science.

Bandura, A. (1969). *Principles of behavior modification.* New York: Holt.

Baratz, S., & Baratz, J. (1970). Early childhood intervention: The social science base of institutional racism. *Harvard Educational Review, 40,* 29–50.

Baron, J. (1981). Reflective thinking as a goal of education. *Intelligence, 5,* 291–309.

Baron, J. (1982). Personality and intelligence. In R. J. Sternberg (Ed.), *Handbook of human intelligence.* New York: Cambridge University Press.

Barona, A., & Santos de Barona, M. (1987). A model for assessment of Limited English Proficient students referred for special education services. In S. H. Fradd and W. J. Tikunoff (Eds.), *Bilingual education and bilingual special education: A guide for administrators* (pp. 183–208). San Diego, CA: College Hill Press.

Barona, A., Santos de Barona, Flores, A. A., & Gutierrez, M. H. (1990). Critical issues in training school psychologists to serve minority school children. In A. Barona & E. Garcia (Eds.), *Children at risk: Poverty, minority status and other issues in educational equity* (pp. 187–200). Washington, DC: National Association of School Psychologists.

Beckles, H. (1989). *White servitude and black slavery in Barbados.* Knoxville: University of Tennessee Press.

Benedict, F. (1959). *Race: Science and politics.* New York: Viking.

Bereiter, C., & Englemann, (1966). *Teaching disadvantaged children in preschool.* Englewood Cliffs, NJ: Prentice-Hall.

Bereton, B. (1985). *Social life in the Caribbean: 1838–1938.* London: Heisman Kingston.

Betancourt, H., & Lopez, S. R. (1993). The study of culture, ethnicity and race in American psychology. *American Psychologist, 48(6),* 629–637.

Bernal, M. (1991, October). Jamaica today. *American Visions, Special Issue,* 2–6.

Bernal, M. E., & Padilla, A. M. (1982). Status of minority curricula and training in clinical psychology. *American Psychologist, 37,* 780–787.

Berry, J. (1980). Cultural universality of any theory of human intelligence remains an open question. *Behavioral and Brain Sciences, 3,* 584–585.

Berry, J. W., Kim, U., Minde, T., Kim, U., Mok, D. (1987). Comparative studies of acculturative stress. *International Migration Review, 21(3)*, 491–511.

Bersoff, D. N. (1981). Testing and the law. *American Psychologist, 36*, 1047–56.

Berzonsky, M. (1971). The role of familiarity in children's explanations of physical causality. *Child Development, 42*, 705–715.

Binet, A., & Simon, T. (1905). Methods nouvelles pour le diagnostic du niveau intellectual des anormaux. *L'Annee psychologique, 11*, 245–336.

Black, F. W. (1973). Reversal and rotation errors by normal and retarded readers. *Perceptual Motor Skills, 36*, 895–898.

Blair, S., Blair, M., & Madamba, A. (1999). Racial/ethnic differences in high school students' academic performance: Understanding the interweave of social class and ethnicity in the family. *Journal of Comparative Family Studies, Vol. 30*, 539–642.

Boehm (1971). *Boehm test of basic concepts.* New York: The Psychological Corporation.

Bogen, E. (1990). *Caribbean immigrants in New York City.* New York, NY: New York City Planning Division, Office of Immigrant Affairs.

Borely, C., & Simmons, H. (1987). *English for CXC.* Surrey: Nelson Caribbean.

Borowski, J. G., & Maxwell, S. E. (1985). Looking for Mr. Good-g: General intelligence and processing speed. *The Behavioral and Brain Science, 8(2)*, 221–222.

Bourdieu, P., & Passeron, J. C. (1977). *Reproduction in education, society and culture.* Beverly Hills, CA: Sage.

Bowen, M. (1978). *Family therapy in clinical practice.* New York: Jason Aronson.

Boyd, D. (1996). Dominance concealed through diversity: Implications of inadequate perspectives on cultural pluralism. *Harvard Educational Review, 66(3)*, 609–630.

Boyd-Franklin, N. (1989). *Black families in therapy.* New York: Guilford Press.

Boykin, A. W. (1979). Psychological behavioral verve: Some theoretical explorations and empirical manifestations. In A. W. Boykin, A. J. Franklin, & J. F. Yates (Eds.), *Research directions of Black psychologists* (pp. 351–367). New York: Russell Sage Press.

Boykin, A. W., & Allen, B. (1988). Rhythmic movement facilitation of learning in working class Afro-American children. *Journal of Genetic Psychology, 149*, 335–348.

Boykin, A. W., & Allen, B. (1992). African-American children and the educational process: Alleviating cultural discontinuity through prescriptive pedagogy. *School Psychology Review, 21(4)*, 586–596.

Boykin, A. W., (1983). The academic performance of Afro-American children. In J. T. Spence (Ed.), *Achievement and achievement motives* (pp. 322–371). San Francisco: Freeman.

Bracken, B. A. (1986). Incidence of basic concepts in the directions of five commonly used American tests of intelligence. *School Psychology International, 7*, 1–10.

Bracken, B. A., & Barona, A. (1991). State of the art procedures for translating, validating and using psychoeducational tests in cross-cultural assessment. *School Psychology International, 12*, 119–132.

Braden, J. P. (1995). For whom the bell tolls: Why the bell curve is important for school psychologists. *School Psychology Review, 24(1)*, 27–35.

Bradley, R. H., Caldwell, B. M., Rock, S. L., Ramey, C. T., Barnard, K. E., Gray, C., Gottfried, A. W., Mitchell, S., Hammond, M., Siegel, L. S., & Johnson, D. (1988). Home environment and cognitive development in the first three years of life: A collaborative study involving six sites and three ethnic groups in North America. *Developmental Psychology, 25*, 217–235.

Bradley, R., Caldwell, B., & Rock, S. (1988). Home environment and school performance: A ten year follow-up and examination of three models of environmental action. *Child Development, 59*, 85.

Brand, C. R., & Deary, I. J. (1982). *Intelligence and "inspection time." A model for intelligence.* Berlin: Springer Verlag.

Brannigan, G. G., & Brunner, N. A. (1989). *The modified version of the Bender gestalt test for pre-school and primary school children*. Brandon, VT: Clinical Psychology Publications.

Brannigan, G. G., & Brunner, N. A. (1992). Comparison of the qualitative and developmental scoring systems for the modified version of the Bender gestalt test. *Journal of School Psychology, 31*, 327–330.

Brice, J. (1982). West Indian families. In M. McGoldrick, J. K. Pearce, & J. Giordana (Eds.), *Ethnicity and family therapy* (pp. 123–133). New York: Guilford Press.

Brice-Baker, J. (1996). Jamaican families. In M. McGoldrick, J. Pearce, & J. Giordano (Eds.), *Ethnicity and family therapy* (2nd ed.). New York: Guilford Press.

Brice Heath, S. (1989). Oral and literate traditions among Black Americans living in poverty. *American Psychologist, Vol. 44, No. 2*, 367–373.

Brislin, R. W. (1970). Back translation for cross-cultural research. *Journal of Cross Cultural Psychology, 1*, 185–216.

Brislin, R. W. (1980). Translation and content analysis of oral and written materials. In H. C. Triandis & J. W. Berry (Eds.), *Methodology: Handbook of cross-cultural psychology* (Vol. 2) (pp. 389–444). Boston, MA: Allyn and Bacon.

Brislin, R. W. (1986). The wording and translation of research instruments. In W. J. Lonner & J. W. Berry (Eds.), *Field methods in cross-cultural research* (pp. 137–164). Beverly Hills, CA: Sage.

Brody, J. (1996) Aggressiveness and delinquency in boys is linked to lead in bones. *New York Times, Health Section K*, p. 4.

Bronfenbrenner, V. (1977). Towards an experimental ecology of human development. *American Psychologist, 45*, 513–530.

Brown, M. T., & Landrum-Brown, J. (1995). Counselor supervision: Cross-cultural perspectives. In J. G. Ponterotto, J. M. Casas, L. A. Suzuki, & C. M. Alexander (Eds.), *Handbook of multi-cultural counseling* (pp. 263–286). California: Sage Publications.

Bruner, J. S. (1983). *Child's talk*. New York: Norton.

Bruner, J. S., Olver, R. R., & Greenfield, P. M. (1966). *Studies in cognitive growth*. New York: Wiley.

Budman, C., Lipson, J., & Meleis, A. (1992). The cultural consultant in mental health care: The case of an Arab adolescent. *American Journal of Orthopsychiatry, 62*, 359–370.

Burdoff, M. (1987a). The validity of learning potential assessment. In C. S. Lidz (Ed.), *Dynamic assessment: An interactional approach to evaluating learning potential*, New York: Guilford Press.

Burke, J., & Tompkins, D. (1991, October). Reggae powerful journey. *American Visions, Special Issue*, 10–11.

Burnam, M. A., Hough, R. L., Kamo, M., Escobar, J. I., & Telles, C. A. (1987). Acculturation and lifetime prevalence of psychiatric disorders among Mexican Americans in Los Angeles. *Journal of Health and Social Behavior, 28*, 89–102.

Butcher, J. N. (1982). Cross-cultural research methods in clinical psychology. In P. C. Kendall & J. N. Butcher (Eds.). *Handbook of research methods in clinical psychology*, (pp. 273–308). New York: John Wiley.

Butcher, J. N., & Graham, J. R. (1994). The MMPI-2: A new standard for personality assessment and research in clinical settings. *Measurement and Evaluation in Counseling and Development, 27*, 131–150.

Calvert, M. B., & Murray, S. L. (1985). Environmental Communication Profile: An assessment procedure. In C. S. Simon (Ed.), *Communication skills and classroom success: Assessment of language disabled students* (pp. 135–165).

Carey, S. (1985). *Conceptual change in childhood*. Cambridge: MIT Press.

Carlson, J. S. (1985). The issue of g: Some relevant questions. *The Behavioral and Brain Science, 8(2)*, 224–225.

Carney, C. G., & Kahn, K. B. (1984). Building competencies for effective cross-cultural counseling: A developmental view. *The Counseling Psychologist, 12(1)*, 111–119.

Carr, T. H., & McDonald, J. L. (1985). Different approach to individual differences. *The Behavioral and Brain Science, 8(2),* 225–227.

Carraher, T. N., Carraher, D., & Schliemann, A. D. (1985). Mathematics in the streets and in schools. *British Journal of Development Psychology, 3,* 21–29.

Carroll, J. B. (1961). Fundamental considerations in testing for English proficiency of foreign students. In *Testing the English proficiency of foreign students* (pp. 31–40). Washington, D.C.: Center for Applied Linguistics.

Carroll, J. B. (1993). *Human cognitive abilities.* Cambridge: Cambridge University Press.

Carrow, E. (1974). *Carrow Elicited Language Inventory.* Boston: Teaching Resources.

Carter, R. (1995). *The influence of race and racial identity in psychotherapy.* New York: John Wiley & Sons.

Casas, J. M., & Casas, A. (1994). *Acculturation: Theory, models, and Implications.* Santa Cruz, CA: Network.

Casas, J. M., Ponterotto, J. G., & Gutierrez, J. M. (1986). An ethical indictment of counseling research and training: The cross-cultural perspective. *Journal of Counseling and Development, Vol. 64, January,* 347–349.

Cattell, R. B. (1963). Theory of fluid and crystallized intelligence: A critical experiment. *Journal of Educational Psychology, 54,* 1–22.

Cattell, R. B. (1973). *Technical supplement for the Culture Fair Intelligence tests Scales 2 and 3,* Champaign, ILL: Institute for Personality and Ability Testing.

Cavalli-Sforza, L., Menozzi, P., & Piazza, A. (1994). *The history and geography of human genes.* New Jersey: Princeton University Press.

Ceci, S. (1990). *On intelligence: More or less.* New Jersey: Prentice Hall.

Chappell, G. E. (1980). Oral language performance of upper elementary school students obtained via story reformulation. *Language, Speech and Hearing Services in Schools, 11,* 236–251.

Charles, E. (1991). Effecting a regional plan for progress. *Caribbean Affairs, 4(2),* 25–30.

Chi, M. T. H. (1978). Knowledge structures and memory development. In R. S. Siegler (Ed.), *Children's thinking: What develops?* Hillsdale, NJ: Lawrence Erlbaum.

Chon, M. (1995). The truth about Asian Americans. In R. Jacoby & N. Glauberman (Eds.). *The bell curve debate* (pp. 238–240). New York: Random House.

Christensen, E. (1975). Counseling with Puerto Ricans: Some cultural considerations. *Personnel and Guidance Journal, 53(5),* 349–356.

Christiansen, J., Thornley-Brown, A., & Robinson, J. (1984). *West Indians in Toronto.* Toronto, Canada: Family Service Association of Metropolitan Toronto.

Chomsky, N. (1956). Three models for the description of language. In I. R. E. *Transactions on Information Theory*, Vol. IT-2 (pp. 113–124).

Clark, C. (1971). The significance of soul. *Contemporary Psychology, 16(1),* 11–12.

Clark, C. (1975). The Shockley–Jensen thesis: A contextual appraisal. *The Black Scholar, July–August,* 3–11.

Clarke, D. (1991). *The impact of foreign born inmates on the New York State Department of Correctional Services* (pp. 1–16). Division of Program Planning, Research and Education, the State Office Building Campus.

Clarke, K. B., & Clarke, M. P. (1947). *Racial identification and preferences in Negro children: Readings in Social Psychology.* New York: Holt and Company.

Clarke, V., & Bolarinde, O. (1989). *Adjustment of Caribbean immigrants in New York: Social and economic dimension.* New York: Caribbean Research Center.

Coelho, E. (1976). West Indian students in the secondary schools. *TESL Talk, 7(4),* 37–46.

Coelho, E. (1976). West Indian students in the secondary schools. *TESL Talk, 7(4),* 37–46.

Coelho, E. (1991). *Caribbean students in Canadian schools.* Toronto: Pippin.

Coelho, E. (1991). *Caribbean students in Canadian schools.* Ontario, Canada: Pippin Publishing Ltd.

Cohen, R. (1969). Conceptual styles, culture conflict, and non-verbal tests of intelligence. *American Anthropologist, 71(5),* 828–857.

College Entrance Examination Board. (1985). *National college bound seniors, 1985.* New York: College Entrance Examination Board.

Cohen, Y. A. (1956). Structure and function: Family organization and socialization in a Jamaican community. *American Anthropologist, 58,* 664–680.

Cohen, J. (1993). Moral pluralism and political consensus. In D. Copp, J. Hamilton, & J. E. Roemer (Eds.), *The idea of democracy* (pp. 270–291). Cambridge, Eng.: Cambridge University Press.

Collins, P. H. (1991). *Black feminist thought: Knowledge, consciousness, and the politics of empowerment.* New York: Routeledge.

Comer, J., Haynes, N., Joyner, E., & Ben-Avie, M. (Eds.) (1996). *Rallying the whole village: The Comer process for reforming education.* New York: Teachers College, Columbia University Press.

Connelly, J. B. (1983). Comparative analysis of two tests of visual-fine motor integration among Indian and Non-Indian children. *Perceptual and Motor Skills, 57,* 1079–1082.

Courtland, L., & Thomas, A. (1983). Rural minority adolescents: New focus in career counseling. Paper presented at the annual convention of the American Psychological and Guidance Association, Washington, DC: March.

Craig, D. (1966). Teaching English to Jamaican Creole speakers: A model of a multi-dialect situation. *Language Learning, 16 (1&2),* 49–61.

Cronbach, L. J. (1975). Five decades of public controversy over mental testing. *American Psychologist, January,* 1–14.

Cuellar, L., Arnold, B., & Maldonado, R. (1995). Acculturation Rating Scale for Mexican Americans – 11: A revision of the original ARSMA scale. *Hispanic Journal of Behavioral Sciences, 17,* 275–304.

Cummins, J. (1984). *Bilingualism and special education: Issues in assessment and pedagogy.* San Diego: College Hill Press.

Cummins, J., & Laquerre, M. (1990). Visual-motor assessment. In C. Reynolds & R. Kamphus (Eds.), *Handbook of psychological and educational assessment of children: Intelligence and achievement* (pp. 593–610). New York: The Guilford Press.

Cummins, J. (1989). A theoretical framework for bilingual special education. *Exceptional Children, Vol. 56, No. 2,* 111–119.

Damico, J. S. (1991). Descriptive assessment of communicative ability in limited English proficient students. In. E.V. Hamayan & J.S. Damico (Eds.), *Limiting bias in the assessment of bilingual students.* Austin, Texas: pro.ed.

Damico, J. S. (1985). *The effectiveness of direct observation as a language assessment technique.* Albuquerque, NM: University of New Mexico. Unpublished doctoral dissertation.

Damico, J. S., & Oller, J. W. (1985). *Spotting language problems.* San Diego: Los Amigos Research Associates.

Dana, R. (Ed.) (2000). *Handbook of cross-cultural and multicultural personality assessment.* Mahwah, NJ: Lawrence Erlbaum Associates.

Dana, R. H. (1993). *Multicultural assessment perspectives for professional psychology.* Boston: Allyn & Bacon.

Daniel, E. (1952). *West Indian histories* (Vol. 1–3). London: Thomas Nelson & Sons.

Darling-Hammond, L. (1994). Performance-based assessment and educational equity. *Harvard Educational Review, Vol. 64, No. 1,* 5–30.

Darling-Hammond, L., & Goodwin, L. (1993). Progress toward professionalism in teaching. In G. Kawelti (Ed.), *Challenges and achievements of American education* (pp. 19–52). Alexandria, VA: Association for Supervision and Curriculum Development.

Das, J. P. (1985). Interpretations for a class on minority assessment. *The Behavioral and Brain Science, 8(2),* 228–229.

Das, J. P., Naglieri, J., & Kirby, J. (1994). *Assessment of cognitive processes.* Boston, MA: Allyn and Bacon.

Day, J. D. (1983). The zone of proximal development. In M. Pressley & J. R. Levin (Eds.), *Cognitive strategy research: Psychological foundations* (pp. 155–176). New York: Springer-Verlag.

De Albuquerque, K. (1979). The future of the Rastafarian movement. *Caribbean Review, 8(4),* 22.

De Avila, E. (1974). The testing of minority children—A neo-Piagetian approach. *Today's Education, November–December,* 72–75.

De Avila, E. (1976). Mainstreaming ethnically and linguistically different children: An exercise in paradox or a new approach. In R. L. Jones (Ed.), *Mainstreaming and the minority child* (pp. 65–76). Reston, VA: Council for Exceptional Children.

Dean, R. S. (1986). Perspective on the future of neuropsychological assessment. In B. S. Plake & J. C. Witt (Eds.), *Buros series on measurement and testing: Future of testing and measurement* (pp. 310–330). Hillsdale, NJ: Erlbaum.

Deutch, M. (1965). The role of social class in language development and cognition. *American Journal of Orthopsychiatry, 35,* 78–88.

DeFour, D. (1991). Issues in mentoring ethnic minority students. *Focus, 5(1),* 1–2.

deHirsch, K., Jansky, J., & Langford, S. W. (1986). *Predicting reading failure.* New York: Harper & Row Publishers.

Delahunty, R. (1988). Perspectives on within group scoring. Special issue: Fairness in employment testing. *Journal of Vocational Behavior, Vol. 33(3),* 463–477.

Delgado-Gaitan, C. (1987). Traditions and transitions in the learning process of Mexican children: An ethnographic view. In G. Spindler & L. Spindler (Eds.), *Interpretative ethnography of education: At home and abroad* (pp. 333–359). Hillsdale, NJ: Erlbaum

Dillard, J. M. (1983). *Multicultural counseling.* Chicago: Nelson Hall.

Domokos-Cheng Ham, M. A. (1989). Empathetic understanding: A skill for joining with immigrant families. *Journal of Strategic and Systemic Therapies, 8(2),* 36–40.

Domokos-Cheng Ham, M. A. (1989). Family therapy with immigrant families: Constructing a bridge between different world views. *Journal of Strategic and Systemic Therapies, 8,* 1–13.

Draguns, J. (1973). Comparisons of psychopathology across cultures. *Journal of Cross Cultural Psychology, March,* 9–47.

Draguns, J. G. (1987). Psychological disorders across cultures. In P. Pedersen (Ed.), *Handbook of cross-cultural counseling and therapy* (pp. 55–62). New York: Praeger.

Dressler, W. (1985). Stress and sorcery in three social groups. *International Journal of Social Psychiatry, 31(4),* 275–281.

Duckworth, J., & Anderson, W. (1995). *MMPI and MMPI-2: Interpretation for counselors and clinicians (4th ed.).* Bristol, PA: Accelerated Development.

Dumas, J. (1989). *Current demographic analysis of Caribbean immigrants in Canada.* Ottawa: Caribbean Government Publishing Center.

Dunn, L. M., & Dunn, L. M. (1982). *Peabody picture vocabulary test.* Circle Pines, MN: American Guidance Service.

Dunn, R. (1978). *Teaching students through their individual learning styles: A practical approach.* Reston, VA: Reston Publishing Co., Division of Prentice Hall.

Dunn, R., Gemake, J., Jalali, F., & Zenhausern, R. (1990). Cross cultural differences of elementary age students from four ethnic backgrounds. *Journal of Multicultural Counseling and Development, April,* 18.

Eberhardt, J. L. & Randall, J. L. (1997). The essential notion of race. *American Psychological Society, 8(3),* 198–203

Edwards, V. K. (1979). *The West Indian student in British schools.* London: Routeledge and Kagan Paul.

Edwards, W. F. (1983). Code selection and shifting in Guyana. *Language in Society, 12(3).*

Education Trust (1998). *Education Watch: The education trust state and national data book* Vol. 11. Washington, D.C., The Education Trust.

Elliot-Lewis, M. (1989). Responses to problems experienced by immigrant children. In V. Clarke & B. Obede (Eds.), *Adjustment of Caribbean immigrants in New York: Educational dimensions* (pp. 43–56). New York: Caribbean Research Center.

Ellis, A. (1974). *Humanistic psychotherapy: The rational emotive approach.* New York: McGraw Hill Book Co.

Elliston, I. (1985). Counseling West Indians immigrants: Issues and answers. In R. Samuda & A. Wolfgang (Eds.), *Intercultural counseling and assessment: Global perspective.* Lewiston: Hogrefe International Inc.

Eno, L., & Deitchmann, J. (1980). A review of the Bender gestalt test as a screening instrument for brain damage with school-aged children of normal intelligence since 1970. *The Journal of Special Education, 14,* 37–45.

Erikson, E. (1983). *Childhood and society* (2nd ed.). New York: Norton.

Erikson, E. (1980). *Identity and the life cycle.* New York: W. W. Norton and Company.

Esquivel, G. (1985). *Best practices in the assessment of limited English proficient and bilingual children.* Bilingual School Psychology Program, Fordham University, NY.

Esquivel, G. (1985). Best practices in the assessment of limited English proficient and bilingual children. In A. Thomas & J. Grimes (Eds.), *Best practices in school psychology I* (pp. 113–123). Washington DC: National Association of School Psychologists.

Eysenck, H. J. (1979). *The structure and measurement of intelligence.* Berlin: Springer.

Eysenck, H. J. (1982). Introduction. In H. J. Eysenck (Ed.), *A model for intelligence.* Berlin: Springer Verlag.

Fabrega, H. (1969). Social psychiatric aspects of acculturation and migration. *Comprehensive Psychiatry, 10(4),* 314–326.

Fairchild, H. H. (1991). Scientific racism: The cloak of objectivity. *Journal of Social Issues, 47(3),* 101–115.

Falicov, C. (1988). Learning to think culturally in family therapy training. In H. Little, D. Breunlin, & D. Schwartz (Eds.), *Handbook of family therapy training and supervision* (pp. 335–357). New York, NY: Guilford.

Farnham-Diggory, S. (1970). Cognitive synresis in Negro and white children. *Monograph of the Society for Research in Child Development, 35(2),* Serial No. 135.

Feuer, C. H. (1985). The political use of Rasta. *Caribbean Review, 14(4),* 48.

Feuerstein, R. (1979). *The dynamic assessment of retarded performers: The Learning Potential Assessment Device, theory, instruments and techniques.* Baltimore, MD: University Park.

Feuerstein, R., Falik, L. H., & Feuerstein, R. (1998). The Learning Potential Assessment Device: An alternative approach to the assessment of learning potential. In R. J. Samuda, R. Feuerstein, A. S. Kaufman, J. Lewis, R. J. Sternberg & associates (Eds.), *Advances in cross-cultural assessment.* CA: Sage Publications

Fields, S. (1979). Mental health and the melting pot. *Innovations, 6(2),* 2–3.

Figueroa, A. F., Sandoval, J., & Merino, B. (1984). School psychology and limited English proficient children: New competencies. *Journal of School Psychology, 22,* 133–143.

Figueroa, R. A. (1990). Best practices in the assessment of bilingual children. In A. Thomas & J. Grimes (Eds.), *Best practices in school psychology II* (pp. 93–106). Washington DC: National Association of School Psychologists.

Fouad, N., & Hansen, J. (1987). Cross-cultural predictive accuracy of the Strong Campbell Interest Inventory. *Measurement and Evaluation in Counseling and Development, Vol. 20(1),* 3–10.

Fouad, N., Cudeck, R., & Hansen, J. (1984). Convergent validity of the Spanish and English forms of the Strong Campbell Interest Inventory for bilingual Hispanic high school students. *Journal of Counseling Psychology, Vol. 31(3),* 339–348.

Fowers, B. J. & Richardson, F. C. (1997). Why is multiculturalism good? *American Psychologist, 51*, 609–621

Fox, D. (1991). Neuropsychology, achievement and Asian-American culture: Is relative functionalism oriented times three? *American Psychologist, Vol. 46(8)*, 877–878.

Freire, P. (1970). *Pedagogy of the oppressed.* New York: Seabury Press.

Friedman, E. (1982). The Myth of Shiska. In M. McGoldrick, J. K. Pearce, & J. Giordano, J. (Eds.), *Ethnicity and family therapy* (pp. 123–133). New York: Guilford Press.

Frisby, C. L. (1992). Issues and problems in the influence of culture on the psychoeducational needs of African American children. *School Psychology Review, 21(4)*, 532–551.

Frisby, C. L. (1995). When facts and orthodoxy collide: The bell curve and the robustness criterion. *School Psychology Review, 24(1)*, 12–19.

Frostig, M., & Maslow, P. (1973). *Learning problems in the classroom: Prevention and remediation.* New York: Grune & Stratton.

Fuchs, L. S., & Fuchs, D. S. (1990). Curriculum-based Assessment. In C. R. Reynolds & R. W. Kamphaus (Eds.), *Handbook of psychological and educational assessment of children* (pp. 435–455). New York: Guilford Press.

Gamoran, A., Nystrand, M., Berends, M., & Le Pore, P. C. (1995). An organizational analysis of the effects of ability groups. *American Research Journal, 32*, 687–715.

Garcia, G. E., & Pearson, P. D. (1994). Assessment and diversity. In L. Darling-Hammond (Ed.), *Review of research in education, 20* (pp. 337–383). Washington, DC: American Educational Research Association.

Gardner, H. (1992). Assessment in context: The alternative to standardized testing. In B. Gifford & M. C. O'Connor (Eds.), *Changing assessments: Alternative views of aptitude, achievement and instruction* (pp. 77–119). Boston: Kluwer.

Gardner, H. (1983). *Frames of mind: The theory of multiple intelligences.* New York: Basic Books.

Gardner, H. (1993). *Multiple intelligences.* New York: Basic Books.

Gardner, H. (1989). Zero-based arts education: An introduction to Arts PROPEL. *Studies in Art Education, 30*, 71–83.

Gauvain, M. (1995). Thinking in niches: Sociocultural influences on cognitive development. *Human Development, 38*, 25–45

Garrett, H. E. (1961). The equalitarian dogma. *Mankind Quarterly, 1*, 253–257.

Gay, J., & Cole, M. (1967). *The new mathematics and an old culture.* New York: Holt, Rinehart & Winston.

Ghassemzadeh, H. (1988). A pilot study of the Bender Gestalt Test in a sample of Iranian normal children. *Journal of Clinical Psychology, 44(5)*, 787–792.

Gibbs, J. T. G., & Huang, L. N. (1989). *Children of color.* San Francisco: Jossey-Bass Publishers.

Gibson, A. (1985). *A light in the dark tunnel.* London: Caribbean House.

Gibson, A. (1986). *The unequal struggle.* London: Caribbean House.

Gickling, E., & Havertape, J. (1981). *Curriculum-based assessment (CBA).* Minneapolis: National School Psychology Inservice Training Network.

Giles, R. (1977). *The West Indian experience in British schools.* London: Heinemann London.

Gilmore, G., Chandy, J., & Anderson, T. (1975). The Bender-Gestalt and the Mexican American student: A report. *Psychology in the Schools, 12(2)*, 172–175.

Gladstein, G. (1983). Understanding empathy: Integrating counseling, developmental and social psychology perspective. *Journal of Counseling Psychology, 30(4)*, 467–482.

Glaser, R. (1977). *Adaptive education: Individual diversity and learning.* New York: Holt, Rinehart & Winston.

Glaser, R. (1990). Testing and assessment: *O tempora! O mores!* Pittsburgh, PA: University of Pittsburgh, Learning Research and Development Center.

Good, T. & Brophy, J. (1994). *Looking in classrooms* (4th ed.). New York: Harper Collins.

Goodstein, C. (1990). America's cities: The new immigrants in the schools. *Crisis, 98(5),* 17–29.

Gopaul-McNicol, S. (1988). Racial identification and racial preference of black preschool children in New York and Trinidad. *The Journal of Black Psychology, 14(2),* 65–68.

Gopaul-McNicol, S. (1992a). Understanding and meeting the psychological and educational needs of African American and Spanish speaking students. *School Psychology Review, 21(4),* 529–531.

Gopaul-McNicol, S. (1992b). Implications for school psychologists: Synthesis of the miniseries. *School Psychology Review, 21(4),* 597–600.

Gopaul-McNicol, S. (1993). *Working with West Indian families.* New York: Guilford Press.

Gopaul-McNicol, S. (1997). *Multicultural/Multimodal/Multisystems approach in working with culturally different families.* Connecticut: Praeger, Greenwood Publishing Group.

Gopaul-McNicol, S., & Armour-Thomas, E. (1997a). A case study on the bio-ecological approach to intellectual assessment. *Cultural Diversity and Mental Health, Vol. 3, No. 2,* 40–47.

Gopaul-McNicol, S., & Armour-Thomas, E. (1997b). The role of a bio-ecological assessment system in writing a culturally sensitive report: The importance of assessing other intelligences. *Journal of Social Distress and the Homeless, Vol. 6, No. 2,* 127–139.

Gopaul-McNicol, S., & Beckles, N. (1992). *The use of the Bender-Gestalt Visual-Motor Test with West Indian children.* Unpublished manuscript.

Gopaul-McNicol, S., & Brice-Baker, J. (1997). Caribbean Americans. In S. Friedman (Ed.), *Cultural issues in the treatment of anxiety* (pp. 81–101). New York City, NY: Guilford Publications, Inc.

Gopaul-McNicol, S., & Brice-Baker, J. (1998). *Cross-cultural practice: Assessment, treatment and training,* New York City, NY: John Wiley & Sons, Inc.

Gopaul-McNicol, S., & Thomas-Presswood, T. (1998). *Working with linguistic and culturally different children: Innovative educational and clinical approaches.* Boston, MA: Allyn & Bacon.

Gopaul-McNicol, S., Black, K., & Clark-Castro, S. (1997). Introduction: Intelligence testing with minority children. *Cultural Diversity and Mental Health, Vol. 3, No. 2,* 1–4.

Gopaul-McNicol, S., Thomas, T., & Irish, G. (1991). *A handbook for immigrants: Some basic educational and social issues in the United States of America.* New York: Caribbean Research Center.

Gordon, B. M. (1990). The necessity of African-American epistemology for educational theory and practice. *Journal of Education, 172(3),* 88–106.

Gordon, E. W. (1977). Diverse human populations and problems in educational program evaluation via achievement testing. In M. J. Wargo & D. R. Green (Eds.), *Achievement testing of disadvantaged and minority students for educational program evaluation* (pp. 29–40). New York: CTB/ McGraw Hill.

Gordon, E. W. (1984). Mechanisms of learning achievement and learning dysfunction in able and gifted minority students: *A study in attribute treatment interaction.* Unpublished manuscript.

Gordon, E. W. (1988). *Human diversity and pedagogy.* New Haven, CT: Yale University. Institute for social and Policy Studies.

Gordon, E. W. (1995). Toward an equitable system of educational assessment. *Journal of Negro Education, 64(3),* 360–372.

Gordon, E. W. (1999). *Education and justice: A view from the back of the bus.* New York: Teachers College Press.

Gordon, E. W., & Armour-Thomas, E. (1991). Culture and cognitive development. In L. Okagaki & R. J. Sternberg (Eds.), *Directors of development: Influence of the development of children's thinking* (pp. 83–90). Hillsdale, NJ: Lawrence Erlbaum.

Gordon, E. W., & Green, D. (1974). An affluent society's excuses for inequality: developmental, economic and educational. *American Journal of Orthopsychiatry, 44(1),* 4–18.

Gordon, E. W., Miller, F., & Rollock, D. (1990). Coping with communicentric bias in knowledge production in the social sciences. *Educational Researcher, 19(3),* 14–19.

Gordon, G. (1980). Bias and alternatives in psychological testing. *Journal of Negro Education, 49(3),* 350–360.

Gordon, R. A., & Rudert, E. E. (1979). Bad news concerning IQ tests. *Sociology of Education, 52,* 174–190.

Gottfried, A. W. (1984). Issues concerning the relationship between home environment and early cognitive development. In A. W. Gottfried (Ed.), *Home environment and early cognitive development.* London: Academic Press.

Gould, S. (1981). *The mismeasurement of man.* New York: W. W. Norton & Co.

Grier, W., & Cobbs, P. (1968). *Black rage.* New York: Basic Books.

Gushue, G., & Sciarra, D. (1995). Culture and families: A multidimensional approach. In J. Ponterotto, J. Casas, L. Suzuki, & C. Alexander (Eds.), *Handbook of multicultural counseling.* Thousand Oaks, CA: Sage.

Guthrie, R. (1976). *Even the rat was white.* New York: Harper and Row.

Hall, C. C. (1997). Cultural malpractice. *American Psychologist, Vol. 52. No. 6,* 642–651.

Halsell Miranda, A. (1993). Consultation with culturally diverse families. *Journal of Educational and Psychological Consultation, 4(1),* 89–93.

Hamayan, E. V. & Damico, J. S. (1991). Developing and using a second language. In E. V. Hamayan & J. S. Damico (Eds.), *Limiting bias in the assessment of bilingual students* (pp. 39–75). Austin, TX: Pro.Ed.

Hamayan, E., Kwait, J., & Perlman, R. (1985). *Assessment of language minority students: A handbook for educators.* Arlington Heights: IL: Illinois Resource Center.

Hargis, C. H. (1987). *Curriculum-based assessment: A primer.* Springfield, IL: Charles C. Thomas.

Harkness, S. (1990). A cultural model for the acquisition of language: Implications for the innateness debate. *Developmental Psychology, 23(7),* 727–740.

Hartman, A. (1978). Diagrammatic assessment of family relationships. *Social Casework, 59,* 465–476.

Hartman, A., & Laird, J. (1983). *Family centered social work practice.* New York, NY: The Free Press.

Harwood, A. (1981). *Ethnicity and medical care.* Cambridge, MA: Harvard University Press.

Haynes, N. (1995). How skewed is the bell curve? *Journal of Black Psychology, 21(3),* 275–299.

Heath, S. B. (1983). *Ways with words: Language, life, and work in communities and classrooms.* Cambridge, Eng.: Cambridge University Press

Helms, J. (1985). Cultural identity in the treatment process. In P. Pedersen, *Handbook of cross-cultural counseling and therapy.* Connecticut: Greenwood Press.

Helms, J. E. (1989). Eurocentrism strikes in strange places and in unusual ways. *The Counseling Psychologist, 17,* 643–647.

Helms, J. E. (1992). Why is there no study of cultural equivalence in standardized cognitive ability testing? *American Psychologist, 47(9),* 1083–1101.

Helton, G. B., Workman, E. A., & Matuszek, P. A. (1982). *Psychoeducational assessment: Integrating concepts and techniques.* New York: Grune & Stratton.

Henderson, N. D. (1982). Human behavior genetics. *Annual Review of Psychology, 33,* 403–40.

Hendriques, F. (1953). *Family and color in Jamaica.* London: Eyre and Spottiswoode.

Henry, F. (1982). A Note on Caribbean migration to Canada. *Caribbean Review, 11(1),* 38.

Henry, F., & Wilson, P. (1975). Status of women in Caribbean societies: An overview of their social, economic, and sexual roles. *Social and Economic Studies, 24,* 165–198.

Herrnstein, R. J., & Murray, C. (1994). *The bell curve.* New York: The Free Press.

Herron, W., Ramirez, S., Javier, R., & Warner, L. (1997). Cultural attunement and personality. *Journal of Social Distress and the Homeless, Vol. 6, 2,* 175–193.

High achieving Asian American are fastest growing minority. (October, 1985). *Population Today,* pp. 2, 8.

Hilliard, A. (1991). Do we have the will to educate all children? *Educational Leadership, 49(1),* 31–36.

Hilliard, A. (1996). Either a paradigm shift or no mental measurement: The nonscience and the nonsense of the bell curve. *Cultural Diversity and Mental Health, 2(1),* 1–20.

Hilliard, A. G. (1979). Standardization and cultural bias as impediments to the scientific study and validation of "intelligence." *Journal of Research and Development in Education, 12(2),* 47–58.

Hills, H. I., & Strozier, A. L. (1992). Multicultural training in APA approved counseling psychology programs: A survey. *Professional psychology: Research and Practice, Vol. 23, No. 1,* 43–51.

Hinds, D. (1966). *Journey to an illusion.* London: Heinemann.

Holden, R. (2000). Are there promising MMPI substitutes for assessing psychopathology and personality? Review and prospect. In R. Dana (Ed.), *Handbook of cross-cultural and multicultural personality assessment* (pp. 267–292). Mahwah, NJ: Lawrence Erlbaum Associates.

Holland, J. (1990). *Holland Self-Directed Search.* Latz, FL: Psychological Assessment Resources.

Holman, A. (1983). *Family assessment: Tools for understanding and intervention.* Baverly Hills, CA: Sage.

Holtzman, W. H. (1980). Projective techniques. In H. C. Triandis & J. W. Berry (Eds.), *Handbook of cross-cultural psychology, Volume 2: Methodology.* Boston, MA: Allyn & Bacon.

Homel, P., Palif, M., & Aaronson, D. (Eds.). (1987). *Childhood bilingualism: Aspects of linguistic, cognitive and social development.* Hillsdale, NJ: Lawrence Erlbaum.

Hoover, M. R., Politzer, L., & Taylor, O. (1991). Bias in reading test for Black language speakers: A sociolinguistic perspective. In A. G. Hilliard III (Ed.), *Testing African American students* (pp. 81–98). Morristown, NJ: Aaron Press.

Horn, J. L. (1991). Measurement of intellectual capabilities: A review of theory. In K. S. McGrew, J. K. Werder, & R. W. Woodcock (Eds.), *WJ-R technical manual.* Chicago: Riverside.

Hunt, L. (1967). *Immigrants and the youth service.* London: Her Majesty Stationery Office.

Hutt, M. I. (1977). *The Hutt adaptation of the Bender gestalt test (3rd ed.).* New York: Grune and Stratton.

Ibrahim, F. A., Ohnishi, H., & Wilson, R. P. (1994). Career assessment in a culturally diverse society. *Journal of Career Assessment, 2,* 276– 288.

Irish, J. A. & Clay, C. (1995). *Assessment of Caribbean students.* Brooklyn, NY: Caribbean Diaspora Press, Inc.

Ivnik, R., Smith, G., Petersen, R., Boeve, B., Kokmen, E., & Tangalos, E. (2000). Diagnostic accuracy of four approaches to interpreting neuropsychological tests data. *Neuropsychology, 14(2),* 163–177.

Jacobson, E. (1938). *Progressive relaxation.* Chicago: University of Chicago Press.

Jacoby, R., & Glauberman, N. (Eds.) (1995). *The bell curve debate.* New York: Random House.

Jaeger, M. E., & Rosnow, R. L. (1988). Contextualism and its implications for inquiry. *British Journal of Psychology, 79,* 63–75.

James, C. (1990). *Making it.* Oakville: Mosaic Press.

James, C. L. R. (1984). *Party politics in the West Indies.* Trinidad, West Indies: Imprint Caribbean Ltd.

James, S. (1978). When your patient is black West Indian. *American Journal of Nursing, November,* 1908–1909.

Jansky, J. J., Hoffman, M. J., Layton, J., & Sugar, F. (1989). Prediction: A six year follow-up. *Annals of Dyslexia, 39,* 227–246.

Jansky, J., & de Hirsch, K. (1972). *Preventing reading failure.* New York: Harper & Row.

Javier, R., & Herron, W. (Eds.). (1998). *Personality development and psychotherapy in our diverse society.* Northvale, NJ: Jason Aronson Inc.

Jensen, A. R. (1969). How much can we boost IQ and scholastic achievement? *Harvard Educational Review, 39(1),* 1–123.

Jensen, A. R. (1973). *Educability and group differences.* New York: Harper & Row.

Jensen, A. R. (1974). How biased are culture-loaded tests? *Genetic Psychology Monographs, 90,* 185–244.

Jensen, A. R. (1979). Outmoded theory or unconquered frontier? *Creative Science and Technology, 2,* 16–29.

Jensen, A. R., & Whang, P. A. (1994). Speed of accessing arithmetic facts in long term memory: A comparison of Chinese-American and Anglo-American children. *Contemporary Educational Psychology, 19,* 1–12.

Johnson, F. A. (1988). Contributions of anthropology to psychiatry. In H. Goldman, C. Norwalk, Appleton & Lange (Eds.), *Review of psychiatry, 2nd edition* (pp. 167–181). Washington, DC: American Psychiatric Press.

Johnson, S. D. (1982). *The Minnesota, multiethnic counselor education curriculum: The design and evaluation of an intervention for cross-cultural counselor education.* Unpublished doctoral dissertation, University of Minnesota, Minneapolis.

Johnson, S. D. (1987). Knowing that versus knowing how: Towards achieving expertise through multicultural training for counsel: *The Counseling Psychologist, 15,* 320–331.

Johnson, S. D. (1990). Towards clarifying culture, race and ethnicity in the context of multicultural counseling. *Journal of Multicultural Counseling and Development, 18,* 4.

Jones, E. E. (1978). Black–white personality differences: Another look. *Journal of Personality Assessment, 42,* 244–252.

Jones, E. E., & Korchin, S. (Eds.) (1982). *Minority mental health.* Connecticut: Praeger, Greenwood Publishing Group.

Jones, E. E., & Zoppel, C. L. (1979). Personality differences among Blacks in Jamaica and the United States. *Journal of Cross-Cultural Psychology, 10,* 435–456.

Jones, L. V. (1985). Interpreting Spearman's general factor. *The Behavioral and Brain Science, 8(2),* 233.

Justus, J. (1983). West Indians in Los Angeles community and identity. In R. Bryce-Laporte (Ed.), *Caribbean immigration into the United States.* Smithson Institute.

Karr, S. K. (1982). Bender-Gestalt performance of Sierra Leone, West African children from four sub-cultures. *Perceptual and Motor Skills, 55,* 123–127.

Kashani, J. H., Beck, N.C., Heoper, E. W., Fallhi, C., Corcoran, C. M., McAllister, J. A., Rosenberg, T. K., & Reid, J. CF. (1987). Psychiatric disorders in a community sample of adolescents. *American Journal of Psychiatry, 144,* 584–589.

Katz, L. (1991). Cultural scripts: The home-school connection. *Early child development and care, 73,* 95–102.

Kaufman, A. S. (1979). *Intelligence testing with the WISC-R.* New York: John Wiley

Keil, K. C. (1984). Mechanisms of cognitive development and the structure of knowledge. In R. J. Sternberg (Ed.), *Mechanisms of cognitive development.* San Francisco: Freeman.

Kerr, M. (1952). *Personality and conflict in Jamaica.* Liverpool: Liverpool University Press.

Kim, S. C., (1985). Family therapy for Asian Americans: A strategic-structural framework. *Psychotherapy, 22,* 342–348.

Kiselica, M. S. (1991). Reflections on a multicultural internship experience. *Journal of Counseling and Development, Vol. 70, September/October,* 126–130.

Koppitz, E. (1981). The Bender Gestalt and VADS test performance of learning disabled middle school pupils. *Journal of Learning Disabilities, 14,* 96–98.

Koppitz, E. M. (1975). *The Bender Gestalt Test for young children. (Vol. 2).* New York: Grune & Stratton.

Korman, M. (1974). National conference on levels and patterns of professional training in psychology: Major themes. *American Psychologist, 29,* 301–313.

Kozol, J. (1991). *Savage inequalities: Children in American's schools.* New York, NY: Crown Publishers, Inc.

Krashen, S. (1982). *Principles and practice in second language acquisition.* Hayward, CA: Alemany Press.

Kretschmer, R. E. (1991). Exceptionality and the limited English proficient students: Historical and practical contexts. In E. V. Hamayan & J. S. Davico (Eds.), *Limiting bias in the assessment of bilingual students* (pp. 2–38). Austin, TX: Pro-Ed.

Kroeber, A. & Kluckhohn, C. (1952). Culture: A critical review of concepts and definitions. *Papers of the Peabody Museum of American Archaeology and Ethnology*, Harvard University, 47.

Krumboltz, J. (1994). Improving career development theory from a social learning perspective. In M. Savikas & R. William Lent (Eds.), *Convergence in career development theories: Implications for science and practice* (pp. 9–31). Palo Alto: CPP Books.

Kurtz, B. (1989). Individual differences in cognitive and metacognitive processing. In W. Schnelder & F. Weinert (Eds.), *Interactions among aptitudes, strategies and knowledge in cognitive performance*. New York: Springer-Verlag.

La Rosa, D., & Maw, C. E. (1990). *Hispanic education: A statistical portrait 1990*. Washington, DC: National Council of La Raza.

Laboratory of Comparative Human Cognition. (1982). Culture and intelligence. In R. J. Sternberg (Ed.), *Handbook of human intelligence*. New York: Cambridge University Press.

Lacelle-Peterson, M. W., & Riverá, C. (1994). Is it real for kids? A framework for equitable assessment policies for English language learners. *Harvard Educational Review, 64*(1), 55–75.

Laesch, K. B., & van Kleeck, A. (1987). The Cloze test as an alternative measure of language proficiency of children considered for exit from bilingual education. *Language Learning, 37,* 171–189.

LaFromboise, T., Coleman, H., & Gerton, J. (1993). Psychological impact of biculturalism: Evidence and theory. *Psychological Bulletin, 114,* 395–412.

Lamur, H., & Speckmann, J. (1975). *Adaptation of the migrants from the Caribbean in the European and metropolis*. Papers presented at the 34th annual conference of the American Association of Applied Anthropology, Amsterdam, The Netherlands.

Landrine, H., & Klonoff, E. (1994). The African American Acculturation Scale: Development, reliability, and validity. *Journal of Black Psychology, 20,* 104–127.

Lane, C. (1995). Tainted sources. In R. Jacoby & N. Glauberman (Eds.). *The bell curve debate* (pp. 125–139). New York: Random House.

Larson, V. L., & McKinley, N. L. (1987). *Communication assessment and intervention strategies for adolescents*, Eau Claire, WI: Thinking Publications.

Lave, J. (1977). Tailor-made experiments and evaluating the intellectual consequences of apprenticeship training. *The Quarterly Newsletter of the Institute for Comparative Human Development, 1,* 1–3.

Lave, J., Murtaugh, M., & de la Roche, D. (1984). The dialectic of arithmetic in grocery shopping. In B. Rogoff & J. Lave (Eds.), *Everyday cognition: Its development in social context*. Cambridge, MA: Harvard University Press.

Lazarus, A. A. (1976). *Multimodal behavior therapy*. New York: Springer.

Leary, P., & De Albuquerque, K. (1989). The other side of paradise: Race and class in the 1986 Virgin Islands elections. *Caribbean Affairs, 2*(1), 51–64.

Lefley, H. P. (1979). Prevalence of potential falling-out cases among Black, Latin and non-white populations of the city of Miami. *Social Science and Medicine, 13B,* 113–128.

Lefley, H. P. (1986). Evaluating the effects of cross-cultural training: Some research results. In H. P. Lefley & P. B. Pedersen (Eds.), *Cross-cultural training for mental health professionals* (pp. 265–307). Springfield, IL: Charles C Thomas.

Leininger, M. (1969). Witchcraft practices and psychocultural therapy with urban and United States families. *Human Organizations, 32*(1), 73–83.

Leiter, R. G. (1948). *Leiter International Performance Scale,* Chicago: Stoelting.

Lesiak, J. (1984). The Bender visual motor test: Implications for the diagnosis and prediction of reading achievement. *Journal of School Psychology, 22,* 391–405.

Levinson, E., & Brandt, J. (1997). Career development. In G. Bear, K. Minke, & A. Thomas, *Children's needs II: Development, problems and alternatives*. Bethesda, MD: National Association of School Psychologists.

Lewin, K. (1935). *A dynamic theory of personality*. New York: Guilford.

Lewis, G. (1983). *In ten years of CARICOM*. Papers presented at a seminar sponsored by the Inter-American Development Bank, Washington, DC.

Lewis, J. E. (1998). Nontraditional uses of traditional aptitude tests. In R. J. Samuda R. Feuerstein A. S. Kaufman J. Lewis R. J. Sternberg & associates (Eds), *Advances in cross-cultural assessment*. CA: Sage Publications

Lichtenstein, S. (1993). Transition from school to adulthood: Case studies of adults with learning disabilities who dropped out of school. *Exceptional Children, 59(4)*, 336–348.

Lidz, C. S. (1987). *Dynamic Assessment*. New York: Guilford.

Lidz, C. S. (1991). *Practitioner's guide to dynamic assessment*. New York: Guilford Press.

Lidz, C. S. (Ed.). (1987). *Dynamic assessment: An international approach to evaluating learning potential*. New York: Guilford.

Lipsky, D. R., & Gartner, A. (1996). Inclusion, school restructuring, and the remaking of American society. *Harvard Educational Review, 66(4)*, 762–796.

London, C. (1978). Sensitizing New York City teachers to the Caribbean student. In H. La Fontaine (Ed.), *Perspective in bilingual education* (pp. 95–103). New Jersey: Avery Publishing Group.

London, C. (1980). *Teaching and learning with Caribbean students*. ERIC Document Reproduction Service No. Ed 196 977.

London, C. (1983). Crucibles of Caribbean conditions: Factors for understanding for teaching and learning with Caribbean students in American educational settings. *Journal of Caribbean Studies, 2(2&3)*, 182–188.

London, C. (1984). Caribbean turning point thorough education. NOMMP. *The Africana Studies and Research Center Newsletter, February–March*, 1–2.

London, C. (1987). Ethnic composition of New York City schools. In A. Carrasquillo & E. Sandis (Eds.), *Schooling, job opportunities and ethnic mobility among Caribbean youth in the United States* (pp. 27–37). New York: The Equitable.

London, C. (1988). Educational theorizing in an emancipatory context. A case for Caribbean curriculum. *The Journal of Caribbean Studies, 6(2)*, 163–178.

London, C. (1989). *Through Caribbean eyes*. Chesapeake, VA: ECA Associates.

London, C. (1990). Educating young new immigrants: How can United States cope? *International Journal of Adolescence and Youth, 2*, 81–100.

Lonner, W. J. (1981). Psychological tests and intercultural counseling. In P. B. Pedersen, J. G. Draguns, W. J. Lonner, & J. E. Trimbie (Eds.), *Counseling across cultures* (pp. 275–303). Honolulu, HI: East West Center and University of Hawaii.

Lopez, E. C. (1995). Best practices in working with bilingual children. In A. Thomas & J. Grimes (Eds.), *Best practices in school psychology III* (pp. 1111–1121). Washington, DC: National Association of School Psychologists.

Lopez, E. C. & Gopaul-McNicol, S. (1997). *English as a second language children*. An unpublished manuscript.

Lopez, E. C., Lamar, D., & Scully-Demartini, D. (1997). The cognitive assessment of limited English proficiency children: Current problems and practical recommendations. *Cultural Diversity and Mental Health, 3(2)*, 117–130.

Louden, D. (1981). A comparative study of self-concept among minority and majority group adolescents in English multiracial schools. *Ethnic and Racial Studies, 4(2)*.

Lu, F. G., Lim, R. F., & Mezzich, J. E. (1995). Cross-cultural psychiatry. In J. Oldham & M. Riba, *Review of Psychiatry, 14*. (pp. 477–510). Washington, DC: American Psychiatric Press.

Lubin, B., Wallis, R. R., & Paine, C. (1971). Patterns of psychological test usage in the United States: 1935–1969. *Professional Psychology, 2*, 70–74.

Luria, A. R. (1966). *Human brain and psychological processes*. New York: Harper & Row.

Lustig, D., Brown, C., Lott, A., & Larkin, V. (1998). Concurrent validity of the Careerscope career assessment and reporting system. *Vocational Evaluation and Work Adjustment Bulletin, 31*, 28–31.

Lynch, E. W. (1992). From culture shock to cultural learning. In E. W. Lynch & J. Hanson (Eds.), *Children at risk: Poverty, minority status, and other issues in educational equity* (pp. 65–89). Washington, D C: National Association of School Psychologists.

Mabey, C. (1981). Black British literacy. *Education Research, 23(2),* 83–95.

Mabey, C. (1986). Black pupil's achievement in inner city London. *Education Research, 28(3),* 163–173.

Madaus G. F. (1992). A technological and historical consideration of equity issues associated with proposals to change the nation's testing policy. *Harvard Educational Review, Vol. 64 No. 1,* 76–92.

Maingot, A., Parry, J. H., & Phillip, S. (1987). *A short history of the West Indies.* London, England: MacMillan Publishers Ltd.

Maker, C. J. (1992). Intelligence and creativity in multiple intelligences: Identification and Development. *Educating Able Learners, Fall,* 12–19.

Marin, G, & Marin, B. (1991). *Research with Hispanic populations.* Newbury Park, CA: Sage.

Marsella, A. J., Kinzie, D., & Gordon, P. (1973). Ethnic variation in the expression of depression. *Journal of Cross-Cultural Psychology, 4,* 435–458.

Marshall, D. (1982). The history of Caribbean migration: The case of the West Indies. *Caribbean Review, 11(1),* 6–11.

Matarazzo, J. (1992). Psychological testing and assessment in the 21st century. *American Psychologist, August,* 1007–1018.

Matthews, J. (1989, March 25). Aspiring lawyers already finding a way to make a point. *The Washington Post,* p. A3.

Mbiti, J. (1970). *African religions and philosophy.* Garden City, NJ: Anchor.

McGoldrick, M., Pearce, J. K., & Giordano, J. (1982). *Ethnicity and family therapy.* New York: Guilford Press.

McGrew, K. S. (1994). *Clinical interpretation of the Woodcock Johnson Tests of Cognitive Ability–Revised.* Boston: Allyn and Bacon.

McGrew, K. S. (1995). Analysis of the major intelligence batteries according to a proposed comprehensive Gf-Gc framework of human cognitive and knowledge abilities. In D. P. Flanagan, J. L. Genshaft, & P. L. Harrison (Eds.), *Beyond traditional intellectual assessment: Contemporary and emerging theories, tests and issues.* New York, NY: Guilford. Manuscript submitted for publication.

McKenzie, M. (1986). Ethnographic findings on West Indian American clients. *Journal of Counseling Psychology Development, 65,* 40–44.

McMillan, D., & Meyers, C. (1980). Larry P.: An educational interpretation. *School Psychology Review, 9,* 136–48.

McNerney, M. (1979). The Trinidadian Creole speaker: Performance, awareness and attitude. *TEST Talk, 10(1&2),*

McNerney, M. (1980). Teaching English to West Indian students: Developing a comprehensive yet differentiating approach. *TEST Talk, 11(1),* 26–32.

McNicol, M. (1991). *Helping children adjust to a new culture: A child's perspective.* New York: Multicultural Educational & Psychological Services, P.C.

McRae, M. B., & Johnson, S. (1991). Toward training for competence in multicultural counselor education. *Journal of Counseling and Development, 70, September/October,* 131–135.

Medway, F. (1995). Best practices in assisting families who move and relocate. In A. Thomas & J. Grimes (Eds.), *Best practices in school psychology III* (pp. 977–985). Washington, DC: The National Association of School Psychologists.

Meinchenbaum, D. H. (1977). *Cognitive-behavior modification.* New York: Plenum.

Mercer, J. R. (1973). *Labeling the mentally retarded.* Berkeley: University of California Press.

Mercer, J. R. (1978). *System of multicultural pluralistic assessment.* San Antonio, TX: The Psychological Corporation.

Mercer, J. R. (1979). In defense of racially and culturally non-discriminatory assessment. *School Psychology Digest, 8(1),* 89–115.

Messick, S. (1976). Personality consistencies in cognition and creativity. In S. Messick (Ed.), *Individuality in learning* (pp. 4–22). San Francisco: Jossey- Bass.

Messick, S. (1989). Validity. In R. L. Linn (Ed.), *Educational Measurement* (3rd ed., pp. 13–104). New York: Macmillan.

Mezzich, J., Kleinman, A., & Fabrega, H. (Eds.), (1993). *Revised cultural proposals for DSM-IV (Technical Report).* Pittsburgh, PA: NIMH Culture and Diagnosis Group.

Milkman, R. (1978). A simple exposition of Jensen's error. *Journal of Educational Statistics, 3(3),* 203–208.

Miller, E. L. (1967). *A study of body image, its relationship to self-concept, anxiety and certain social and physical variables in a selected group of Jamaican adolescents.* Unpublished master's thesis, University of the West Indies, Kingston, Jamaica.

Miller-Jones, D. (1989). Culture and testing. *American Psychologist, 44,* 360–366.

Milner, D. (1983). *Children and race.* London: Sage Publications.

Minuchin, S. (1974). *Families and family therapy.* Cambridge, MA: Harvard University Press.

Minuchin, S., Montalvo, B., Guerney, B. G., Jr., Rosman, B. L., & Schumer, F. (1967). *Families of the slums.* New York: Basic Books.

Mio, J. S. (1989). Experiential involvement as an adjunct to teaching cultural sensitivity. *Journal of Multicultural Counseling and Development, 17,* 38–46.

Mollica, R. F., Wyshak, G., & Lowelle, J. (1987). The psychosocial impact of war trauma and torture on Southeast Asian refugees. *American Journal of Psychiatry, 144(12),* 1567–1572.

Moon, J. D. (1993). *Constructing community: Moral pluralism and tragic conflicts.* Princeton, NJ: Princeton University Press.

Morrow, R. (1987). Cultural differences: Be aware. *Academic Therapy, 23(2),* 143–149.

Mosley-Howard, S. (1995). Best practices in considering the role culture. In A. Thomas & J. Grimes (Eds.), *Best practices in school psychology III* (pp. 337–345). Washington DC: National Association of School Psychologists.

Mowder, B. (1980). A strategy for the assessment of bilingual handicapped children. *Psychology in the Schools, 17(1),* 7–11.

Murray, B. (1996). Developing phoneme awareness through books. *Reading and writing: An interdisciplinary Journal, 8(4),* 307–322.

Murray, H. A. (1938). *Explorations in personality.* New York: Oxford University Press.

Murrone, J., & Gynther, M. (1991). Teachers' implicit "theories" of children's intelligence. *Psychological Reports, 69,* 1195–1201.

Murtaugh, M. (1985). The practice of arithmetic by American grocery shoppers. *Anthropology and Education Quarterly, Fall.*

Myers, L. J. (1991). Expanding the psychology of knowledge optimally: The importance of worldview revisited. In R. L. Jones (Ed.), *Black psychology* (3rd ed., pp. 15–28). Berkeley, CA: Cobb & Henry.

National Commission on Teaching (1996). *What matters most: Teaching for America's future.* New York: Author.

Neale, M. D., & McKay, M. F. (1985). Scoring the Hender gestalt test using the Koppitz developmental system: Interrater reliability, item difficulty, and scoring implications. *Perceptual and Motor Skills, 61,* 627–636.

Neisser, U. (1979). The concept of intelligence. *Intelligence, 3,* 217–227.

New York City Police Department. (1985). Rasta crime. *Caribbean Review, 14(1),* 12.

New York City Police Department—Office of Immigrant Affairs and Population Analysis Division (1985, May 11). *Caribbean immigrants in New York City: A demographic summary.* Unpublished manuscript presented to the Caribbean Research Center.

Newmann, F. M., & Wehlagen, G. G. (1995). *Successful school restructuring: A report to the public and educators by the Center on Organization and Restructuring of Schools.* Madison, WI: Wisconsin Center for Education Research.

Newmann, F. M., Marks, H. M., & Gamoran, A. (1995). *Authentic pedagogy and student perform-ance*. Madison, WI: Wisconsin Center for Education Research.

Nichols, J., Cheung, P. C., Lauer, J., & Patashnick, M. (1989). Individual differences in academic motivation: Perceived ability, goals, beliefs and values. *Learning and Individual Differences, 1,* 63–84.

Nichols, R. (1981). Origins, nature and determinants of intellectual development. In M. Begab, H. C. Haywood, & H. Garber (Eds.), *Psychosocial determinants of retarded performance* (Vol. 1). Baltimore: University Park Press.

Noble, C. E. (1969). Race, reality and experimental psychology. *Perspectives in Biology and Medicine, 13,* 10–30.

Nystrand, M. & Gamoran, A. (1988). *A study of instruction as discourse*. Madison, WI: Wisconsin Center for Education Research.

Oakes, J. (1985). *Keeping track: How schools structure inequality*. New Haven, CT: Yale University Press.

Oakes, J. (1990). *Multiplying inequalities. The effects of race, socioeconomic status and tracking on opportunities to learn mathematics and science*. Santa Monica, CA: The Rand Corporation.

Oakland, T. (1977). *Psychological and educational assessment of minority children*. New York: Brunner/Mazel.

Oakland, T. (1995). The bell curve: Some implications for the discipline of school psychology and the practices of school psychology. *School Psychology Review, 24(1),* 20–26.

Oakland, T., & Feigenbaum, D. (1979). Multiple sources of test bias on the WISC-r and Bender gestalt test. *Journal of Consulting and Clinical Psychology, 47(5),* 968–974.

Oakland, T., & Phillips, B. N. (1973). *Assessing minority group children*. New York: Behavioral Publications.

Oberg. (1972). Model for culture shock. *The Personnel and Guidance Journal, February,* 376–378.

Ochs, E. & Schiefflin, B. (1984). Language acquisition and socialization: Three developmental sto-ries and their implications. In R. Shweder & R. LeVine (Eds.), *Culture and its acquisition*. Chicago: University of Chicago Press.

Ogbu, J. U. (1978). *Minority education and caste*. Orlando, FL: Academic Press.

Ogbu, J. U. (1987). Variability in minority responses to schooling: Nonimmigrants vs. immigrants. In G. Spindler (Ed.), *Interpretive ethnography of education at home and abroad* (pp. 255–278). Hillsdale, NJ: Lawrence Erlbaum.

Ogbu, J. U. (1988). Black education: A cultural-ecological perspective. In H. P. McAdoo (Ed.), *Black families* (pp. 169–184). Newbury Park: Sage Publishers.

Oldham, J., & Riba, M. (Eds.) (1995). *Review of psychiatry, Vol. 14,* Washington, DC: American Psychiatric Press. Inc.

Oller, J. W., Jr. (1989). Conclusions toward a rational pragmatism. In J. W. Oller, Jr. (Ed.), *Language and experience: Classic pragmatism* (pp. 223–250). Lanham, MD: University Press of America.

Oller, J. W. & Damico, J. S. (1991). Theoretical considerations in the assessment of LEP students. In. E.V. Hamayan & J.S. Damico (Eds.), *Limiting bias in the assessment of bilingual students*. Austin, Texas: Pro.Ed.

Padilla, A. M. (1979). Critical doctors in the testing of Hispanic Americans: A review and some suggestions for the future. In R. W. Tyler & S. H. White (Eds.), *Testing, teaching and learn-ing: Report of a conference on testing*. Washington, DC: U.S. Government Printing Office.

Palmer, D., Hughes, J., & Juarez, L. (1991). School psychology training and the education of at-risk youth: The Texas A & M university program emphasis on handicapped Hispanic children and youth. *School Psychology Review, 21, No. 4,* 603–616.

Parker, R., & Schaller, J. (1996). Issues in vocational assessment and disability. In E. Szymanski & R. Parker (Eds.), *Work and disability: Issues and strategies in career development and job place-ment* (pp. 127–164). Austin, TX: Pro-Ed.

Parker, W. M., Valley, M. M., & Geary, C. A. (1986). Acquiring cultural knowledge for counselors in training: A multifaceted approach. *Counselor Education and Supervision, 26,* 61–71.

Parry, J., Sherlock, P., & Maingot, A. (1987). *A short history of the West Indies, 4th edition.* London: MacMillan Publishers Ltd.

Parsons, L., & Lawner Weinberg, S. (1993). The Sugar scoring system for the Bender Gestalt Test: An objective approach that reflects clinical judgment. *Perceptual Motor Skills, 77,* 883–893.

Parsons, L., & Weinberg, S. L. (1993). The Sugar scoring system for the Bender gestalt test: An objective approach that reflects clinical judgment. *Perceptual and Motor Skills, 77,* 883–893.

Pasternak, M. (1986). *Helping kids learn multicultural concepts: A handbook of strategies.* Illinois: Research Press Company.

Payne, M. (1989). Use and abuse of corporal punishment: A Caribbean view. *Child Abuse and Neglect, 13,* 389–401.

Pedersen, P. (1987). *Handbook of cross cultural counseling and therapy.* Westport, CT: Greenwood Press.

Pedersen, P. (1995). Culture-centered ethical guidelines for counselors. In J. G. Ponterotto, J. M. Casas, L. A. Suzuki, & C. M. Alexander (Eds.), *Handbook of multicultural counseling* (pp. 34–49). California: Sage Publications.

Pedersen, P. (1995). Culture-centered ethical guidelines for counselors. In J. G. Ponterotto, J. M. Casas, L. A. Suzuki, & C. M. Alexander (Eds.), *Handbook of multicultural counseling* (pp. 34–52). California: Sage Publications?

Pedersen, P. B. (1973, September). *A cross-cultural coalition training model for educating mental health professionals to function in a multicultural population.* Paper presented at the Ninth International Congress of Ethnological and Anthropological Science, Chicago.

Persell, C. H. (1977). *Education and inequality: The roots and results of stratification in America's schools.* New York: Free Press.

Peterson, C., & McCabe, A. (1983). *Developmental psycholinguistics. Three ways of looking at a child's narrative.* New York: Plenum Press.

Philippe, J., & Romain, J. B. (1979). Indisposition in Haiti. *Social Science and Medicine, 13B,* 129–133.

Phillips, A. S. (1976). *Adolescence in Jamaica.* Jamaica: Jamaica Publishing House.

Phinney, J. S. (1996). When we talk about American ethnic groups, what do we mean? *American Psychologist, 51(9),* 918–927.

Pierre, A. (1986). *New capital arithmetic for the Caribbean.* Kingston, Jamaica: Heinemann Educational Books (Caribbean) Ltd.

Pine, G. J. (1972). Counseling minority groups: A review of the literature. *Counseling and Values, 17,* 35–44.

Plata, M. (1982). *Assessment, placement and programming of bilingual exceptional pupils: A practical approach.* Reston, VA: Council for Exceptional Children.

Plomin, R. (1990). The role of inheritance in behavior. *Science, 248,* 183–188.

Plowden, L. (1967). *The Plowden report: Children and their primary schools.* London: Department of Education and Science and Her Majesty's Stationery Office.

Ponterotto, J. G., & Casas, J. M. (1987). In search of multicultural competencies within counselor education. *Journal of Counseling and Development, 64, April,* 430–434.

Ponterotto, J. G., & Casas, J. M. (1991). *Handbook of racial/ethnic minority counseling research.* Springfield, IL: Charles C. Thomas.

Ponterotto, J. M. Casas, J. M., Suzuki, L. A. & Alexander, C. M. (Eds.). (1995). *Handbook of multicultural counseling* (pp. 312–330). Thousand Oaks, CA: Sage Publications.

Poortinga, Y. H., van de Vijver, F. J. R., Joe, R. C., & Van de Koppel, J. M. H. (1987). Peeling the onion called culture: A synopsis. In C. Kagitcibasi (Ed.), *Growth and progress in cross-cultural psychology* (pp. 22–34). Lisse, The Netherlands: Swets& Zeitlinger.

Prasse, D. P. (1986). Litigation and special education: An introduction. *Exceptional children, 52,* 311–312.

Prasse, D. P., & Reschly, D. J. (1986). Larry P.: A case of segregation, testing, or program efficacy? *Exceptional Children, 52(4),* 333–346.

Quinn, N., & Holland, D. (1987). Culture and cognition. In D. Holland & N. Quinn (Eds.), *Cultural models in language and thought* (pp. 3–42). Cambridge: Cambridge University Press.

Rabbit, P. M. (1985). Oh g Dr. Jensen! or, g-ing up cognitive psychology. *The Behavioral and Brain Science, 8(2),* 238–239.

Ramirez, A. (1985). *Bilingualism through schooling: Cross-cultural education for minority and majority students.* Albany, NY: State University of New York Press.

Ramirez, M., III. (1991). *Psychotherapy and counseling with minorities: A cognitive approach to individual and cultural differences.* New York: Pergamon Press.

Raskin, P. (1985). Identity and vocational development. *New Directions for Child Development, 30,* 25–42.

Raskin, P. (1987). *Vocational counseling: A guide for the practitioner.* New York: Teachers College, Columbia University.

Raspberry, W. (1991, May 14th). Right strategies for wrong countries. *New York Daily News,* p. 35.

Raven, J. C. (1938). *Progressive matrices.* London: Lewis.

Rawls, J. (1993). *Political liberalism.* New York: Columbia.

Reid, J. (1986, February). Immigration and the future of U.S. Black Population. *Population Today, 14,* 6–8.

Resnick, L. B., & Resnick, D. P. (1992). Assessing the thinking curriculum: New tools for educational reform. In B. Gifford & M. C. O'Connor (Eds.), *Changing assessments: Alternative views of aptitude, achievement and instruction* (pp. 37–75). Boston: Kluwer.

Reynolds, C., & Kamphus, R. (1990). *Handbook of psychological and educational assessment of children: Intelligence and achievement.* New York: The Guilford Press.

Richardson, L. (1994, April 6). Minority students languish in special education system. *New York Times,* pp. A1, B7.

Ridley, C. R. (1985). Imperatives for ethnic and cultural relevance in psychology training programs. *Professional Psychology: Research and Practice, 16, No. 5,* 611–622.

Riley, M. K., Morocco, C. C., Gordon, S. M., & Howard, C. (1993). Walking the talk: Putting constructivist thinking into practice of constructivist principles. *Educational Horizons, 71(4),* 187–196.

Rimer, S. (1991, September 16). Between two worlds: Dominicans in New York. *New York Times,* p. B6-L.

Roberts, P. (1988). *West Indians and their language.* London: Cambridge University Press.

Robin, R. W., & Shea, J. D. (1983). The Bender Gestalt visual motor test in Papua, New Guinea. *International Journal of Psychology, 18,* 263–270.

Rodriguez-Fernandez, C. M. (1981). Testing and the Puerto Child: A practical guidebook for psychologists and teachers (Doctoral dissertation, University of Massachusetts).

Rogers, C. (1975). Empathetic: An unappreciated way of being. *The Counseling Psychologist, 5(2),* 2–10.

Rogers, C. (1975). What is Rasta? *Caribbean Review, 7(1),* 9.

Rogers, M., Close Conoley, J., Ponterotto, J., & Wiese, M. J. (1992). Multicultural training in school psychology: A national survey. *School Psychology Review, 21, No. 4,* 603–616.

Rogoff, B. (1978). Spot observations: An introduction and examination. *Quarterly Newsletter of the Institute for Comparative Human Development, 2,* 21–26.

Rogoff, B. (1982). Integrating context and cognitive development. In M. Lamb & A. Brown (Eds.), *Advances in development psychology* (Vol. 2). Hillsdale, NJ: Lawrence Erlbaum.

Rogoff, B. & Chavajay, P. (1995). What's become of research on the cultural basis of cognitive development? *American Psychologist, 50(10),* 859–877.

Ronstrom, A. (1989). Children in Central America: Victims of war. *Child Welfare League of America. 58(2)*, 145–153.

Rosenblatt, A., & Attkisson, C. (1992). Integrating systems of care in California for youth with severe emotional disturbances: A descriptive overview of the California AB377 evaluation project. *Journal of Child and Family Studies, 1,* 93–113.

Rosenthal, R., & Jacobson, L. (1968). *Pygmalion in the classroom.* New York: Holt, Rinehart & Winston.

Rothenberg, J. J. (1990). An outcome study of an early intervention for specific learning disabilities, *Journal of Learning Disabilities, 23(5),* 317–320.

Rothenberg, J. J., Lehman, L. B., & Hackman, J. D. (1979). An individualized learning disabilities program in the regular classroom. *Journal of Learning Disabilities, 12(7),* 72–75.

Rowe, H. (Ed.). (1991). *Intelligence, reconceptualization and measurement.* Australian Council for Education Research, Hillsdale, NJ: Lawrence Erlbaum Associates.

Rueda, R., & Matinez, I. (1992). Fiesta educativa: One community's approach to parent training in developmental disabilities for Latino families. *Journal of the Association of Severe Handicaps, 17(2),* 95–103.

Rueda, R., Cardoza, D., Mercer, J. R., & Carpenter, L. (1984). *An examination of special education decision making with Hispanics first-time referrals inlarge urban school districts.* Los Alamitos, CA: Southwest Regional Lab.

Ruiz, P. (1995). Cross-cultural psychiatry. In J. Oldham & M. Riba, *Review of Psychiatry, Vol. 14.* (pp. 467–476). Washington, DC: American Psychiatric Press.

Saakana, A. S., & Pearse, A. (1986). *Towards the decolonization of the British educational system.* London: Frontline Journal/Karnak House.

Sabnani, H. B., Ponterotto, J. G., & Borodovsky, L. G. (1991). White racial identity development and cross-cultural counselor training: A stage model. *The Counseling Psychologist, 19(1),* 76–102.

Saeki, C., & Borow, H. (1987). Counseling and psychotherapy: East and West. In P. Pedersen (Ed.), *Handbook of cross-cultural counseling and therapy* (pp. 223–229). New York: Praeger.

Samuda, R. (1975). From Ethnocentrism to a multicultural perspective in educational testing. *Journal of Afro-American Issues, 3(1),* 4–17.

Samuda, R. (1976). Problems and issues in assessment of minority group children. In R. L. Jones (Ed.), *Mainstreaming and the minority child* (pp. 65–76). Reston, VA: Council for Exceptional Children.

Samuda, R. J., Kong, S. L., Cummins, J., Pascual-Leone, J., & Lewis, J. (1989). *Assessment and placement of minority students.* Lewiston, NY: Hogrefe/ISSP.

Sapp, G. L. (1984). Sociocultural factors and Bender Visual-Motor Gestalt performance. Paper presented at the annual convention of the National Association of School. Psychologists, Pennsylvania.

Sattler, J. M. (1988). *Assessment of children.* San Diego, CA: Jerome M. Sattler Publisher.

Sattler, J. M. (1992). *Assessment of children* (revised and updated 3rd ed.) San Diego, CA: Author.

Sattler, J. M., & Gwynne, J. (1982). Ethnicity and Bender visual motor test performance. *Journal of School Psychology, 20(1),* 69–71.

Saunders, D. R. (1956). Moderator variables in prediction. *Educational and Psychological Measurement, 16,* 209–222.

Savignon, S. (1983). *Communicative competence: Theory and classroom practice* (Texts and contexts in second language teaching). Reading, MA: Addison-Wesley.

Schacter, S., Brannigan, G. G., & Tooke, W. (1991). Comparisons of two scoring systems for the modified revision of the Bender gestalt test. *Journal of School Psychology, 29,* 265–269.

Schaefer, E. S. (1987). Parental modernity and child academic competence: Towards a theory of individual and societal development. *Early Development and Care, 27,* 373–389.

Scheurich, J., & Young, M. (1997). Coloring epistemologies: Are our research epistemologies racially biased? *Educational Researcher, 26(4),* 4–16.

Schmidt, P. (1990, April 18). School reports progress in assessing limited English proficient students. *Education Week, 18,* 1–2.

Scobie, E. (1972). *Black Britannia.* Chicago, IL: Johnson Publishing Company Inc.

Scribner, S. (1986). Thinking in action: Some characteristics of practical thought. In R. Sternberg & R. K. Wagner (Eds.), *Practical intelligence: Nature and origins of competence in the everyday world.* New York: Cambridge University Press.

Semaj, L. (1979). Inside Rasta: The future of a religious movement. *Caribbean Review, 14(1),* 8.

Semel, E., & Wiig, E. (1987). *Clinical evaluation of language fundamentals,* Revised. San Antonio, TX: The Psychological Corporation.

Senior, G. (1997). Interview conducted on 7/11/97 at the Multicultural Educational & Psychological Services, New York.

Separate and unequal. (1993, December 13). *U.S. News & World Report,* pp. 46–60.

Sewell-Coker, B., Hamilton-Collins, J., & Fein, E. (1985). Social work practice with West Indian immigrants. *Social Casework: The Journal of Contemporary Social Work, November,* 563–568.

Shapiro, E. (1990). An integrated model for curriculum based assessment. *School Psychology Review, 19(3),* 331–349.

Shapiro, E. S. (1987). *Behavioral assessment in school psychology.* Hillsdale, NJ: Lawrence Erlbaum Associates.

Shepard, L. (1993). Evaluating test validity. In. L. Darling-Hammond (Ed.), *Review of research in education,* Vol. 19 (pp. 405–450). Washington, DC: American Educational Research Association.

Shepard, L. & Smith, M. L. (1986). Synthesis of research on school readiness and kindergarten retention. *Educational Leadership, 44(3),* 78–86.

Shinn, M. R. (Eds.). (1989). *Curriculum-based measurements: Assessing special children.* New York: Guilford Press.

Shon, S. P., & Ja, D. Y. (1982). Asian families. In M. McGoldrick, J. K. Pearce, & J. Giordano (Eds.), *Ethnicity and family therapy* (pp. 123–133). New York: Guilford Press.

Short, G. (1985). Teacher expectation and West Indian underachievement. *Educational Research, 27(2),* 95–101.

Siegel, L. S. (1984). Home environmental influence on cognitive development in pre-term and full-term children during the first five years. In A. W. Gottfried (Ed.), *Home environment and early cognitive development* (pp. 19234). Orlando, FL: Academic Press.

Silvera, M. (1986). *Silenced.* Toronto: Williams Wallace Production Inc.

Simon, C. S. (1989). *Classroom communication screening procedure for early adolescents: A handbook for assessment and intervention.* Tempe, AZ: Communi-Cog Publications.

Singleton, R. A., Starits, B. C., & Straits, M. M. (1993). *Approaches to social research* (2nd ed.). New York: Oxford University Press.

Slavin, R. E. (1987). *A review of research on elementary ability grouping.* Baltimore, MD: John Hopkins University Press.

Slavin, R. E. (1988). Cooperative learning and student achievement. *Educational Leadership, 45(2),* 31–33.

Sloan, T. S., (1990). Psychology for the third world. *Journal of Social Issues, 46(3),* 1–20.

Skinner, B. F. (1974). *About behaviorism.* New York: Knopf.

Skutnabb-Kangas, T. & Toukomaa, T. (1976). *Teaching migrant children's mother tongue and learning the language of the host country in the context of the sociocultural situation of the migrant family.* Helsinki: The Finnish National Commission for UNESCO.

Snowden, L., & Todman, P. (1982). The psychological assessment of Blacks: New and needed development. In E. E., Jones & S. Korchin (Eds.), *Minority mental health.* Connecticut: Praeger, Greenwood Publishing Group.

Snyder, R. T., Holowenzak, S. P., & Hoffman, N. (1971). A cross-cultural item-analysis of Bender Gestalt protocols administered to ghetto and suburban children. *Perceptual and Motor Skills, 33,* 791–796.

Snyderman, M., & Rothman, S. (1987). Survey of expert opinion on intelligence and aptitude test-ing. *American Psychologist, 42,* 137–144.

Solomon, P. (1992). *Black resistance in high school.* Albany: State University of New York Press.

Soutar-Hynes, M. (1976). West Indian realities in the intermediate grades: The emerging role of the ESD teacher. *TESL Talk, 7(4),* 31–36.

Sowell, T. (1981). *Ethnic America.* New York: Basic Books.

Spearman, C. (1927). *The abilities of man: Their nature and measurement.* New York: Macmillan. (Reprinted 1981, New York: AMS.)

Stanfield, J. (1985). The ethnocentric bias of social science knowledge production. In E. W. Gordon (Ed.), *Review of research in education,* Vol. 12, pp. 387–415.

Stanfield, J. H., II (1993). Epistemological considerations. In J. H. Stanfield II & R. M. Dennis (Eds.), *Race and ethnicity in research methods* (pp. 16–36). Newbury Park, CA: Sage.

Stanfield, J. H., II (1994). Ethnic modeling in qualitative research. In N. K. Denzin & Y. S. Lincoln (Eds.), *Handbook of qualitative inquiry* (pp. 175–188). Newbury Park, CA: Sage.

Sternberg, R. J. (1984). What should intelligence tests test? Implications of a Triarchic theory of intelligence for intelligence testing. *Educational Researcher, January,* 5–15.

Sternberg, R. J. (1985). *Beyond IQ.* New York: Cambridge University Press.

Sternberg, R. J. (1986). *Intelligences applied.* New York: Harcourt Brace Jovanovich, Publishers.

Sternberg, R. J., & Powell, J. S. (1983). Comprehending verbal comprehension. *American Psychologist, 38,* 878–893.

Sternberg, R. J. & Wagner, R. K. (1986). *Practical Intelligence: Nature and origin of competence in the everyday world.* New York Cambridge University Press.

Stetson, B. R. (1934). In C. S. Johnson & S. M. Bond, The investigation of racial differences prior to 1910. *Journal of Negro Education, 39.*

Stewart, R. (1986). *The United States in the Caribbean.* Kingston, London: Heinemann Educational Books Inc.

Strom, R., Johnson, A., Strom, S., & Strom, P. (1992). Designing curriculum for parents of gifted children. *Journal for the Education of the Gifted, 15(2),* 182–200.

Strom, R., Johnson, A., Strom, S., & Strom, P. (1992). Educating gifted Hispanic children and their parents. *Hispanic Journal of Behavioral Sciences, 14(3),* 383–393.

Stroop, J. R. (1935). Studies of interference in serial verbal reactions. *Journal of Experimental Psychology, 18,* 643–661.

Sue, D. W. (1991). A conceptual model for cultural diversity training. *Journal of Counseling and Development, 70,* 99–105.

Sue, D. W. & Sue, D. (1990). *Counseling the culturally different: Theory and practice (2nd ed.).* New York: John Wiley.

Sue, D., Arredondo, P., & McDavis, R. (1992). Multicultural counseling competencies and standards: A call to the profession. *Journal of Multicultural Counseling and Development, 20,* 64–88.

Sue, S. (1981). *Counseling the culturally different.* New York: Wiley.

Sue, S., & Okazaki, S. (1990). Asian-American educational achievements: A phenomenon in search of an explanation. *American Psychologist, 45,* 913–920.

Sue, S., & Zane, N. (1987, January). The role of culture and cultural techniques in psychothera-py. *American Psychologist, 42,* 37–45.

Sugar, F.(1992). A new method for scoring the Bender Gestalt test of visual motor development (unpublished manuscript, The Dalton School, New York, NY).

Super, C. M. (1980). Cognitive development: Looking across at growing up. In C. Super & M. Harkness (Eds.), *New Directions for Child Development: Anthropological Perspectives on Child Development, 8,* 59–69.

Super, D. E. (1987). Career counseling across cultures. In P. Pedersen (Ed.), *Handbook of cross-cul-tural counseling and therapy* (pp. 11–20). Westport, CT: Praeger, Greenwood Publishers.

Super, D. E. (1992a). A comparison of the diagnoses of a graphologist with the results of psychological tests. *Journal of Consulting and Clinical Psychology, 60(3),* 323–326.

Super, D. E. (1992b). Towards a comprehensive theory of career development. In D. Montross and C. Shinkman (Eds.), *Career development: Theory and practice* (pp. 35–64). Springfield, IL: Charles Thomas.

Super, D. E. (1995a). Values: Their nature, assessment and practical use. In D. E. Super, & B. Sverko (Eds.), *Life roles values and careers: International findings of the work importance study* (pp. 54–61). San Francisco, CA: Jossey Bass Social and Behavioral Science Series.

Super, D. E. (1995b). Test of the work importance study model of role salience. In D. E. Super & B. Sverko (Eds.), *Life roles values and careers: International findings of the work importance study* (pp. 321–324). San Francisco, CA: Jossey Bass Social and Behavioral Science Series.

Super, D. E., & Sverko, B. (Eds.) (1995). *Life roles values and careers: International findings of the work importance study.* San Francisco, CA: Jossey Bass.

Supovitz, J. A., & Brennan, R. T. (1997). Mirror, mirror on the wall, Which is the fairest test of all? An examination of the equitability of portfolio assessment relative to standardized tests. *Harvard Educational Review, 67 (3),* pp. 472–502.

Suzuki, D. (1995). Correlation as causation. In R. Jacoby & N. Glauberman (Eds.), *The bell curve debate* (pp. 280–282). New York: Random House.

Suzuki, S. (1969). *Nurtured by love.* New York: Exposition Press.

Swanson, J. (1992). The structure of vocational interest for African American college students. Special Issue: Holland's theory. *Journal of Vocational Behavior, 40(2),* 144–157.

Tapp, J. L., Kelman, H., Triandis, H., Wrightsman, L., & Coelho, G. (1974). Advisory principles for ethical considerations in the conduct of cross-cultural research: Fall 1973 Revision. *International Journal of Psychology, 9,* 231–349.

Taylor, R. (1984). *Assessment of exceptional students: Educational and psychological procedures.* Englewood Cliffs, NJ: Prentice-Hall.

Taylor, R. L., & Partenio, I. (1984). Ethnic differences on the Bender Gestalt: Relative effects of measured intelligence. *Journal of Consulting and Clinical Psychology, 52(5),* 784–788.

Taylor, R. L., Kaufman, D., & Partenio, I. (1984). The Koppitz developmental scoring system for the Bender Gestalt: Is it development? *Psychology in the Schools, 21,* 425–428.

Tharp, R. G. (1989). Psychocultural variables and constants. *American Psychologist. Vol. 44, No. 2,* 349–359.

Thomas, S. (1999). Vocational evaluation in the 21st century. *The Journal of Rehabilitation, 65(1),* 1–10.

Thomas, T. (1991). *Post traumatic stress disorder in children.* Paper presented in August at the annual meeting of the American Psychological Association, Boston, MA.

Thomas, T., & Gopaul-McNicol, S. (1991). *An immigrant handbook on special education in the United States of America.* New York: Multicultural Educational & Psychological Services, P.C.

Thomas, W. B. (1986). Mental testing and tracking for the social adjustment of an urban underclass, 1920–1930. *Journal of Education, 168(2),* 9–30.

Thompson, R. W., & Hixson, P. (1984). Teaching parents to encourage independent problem solving in preschool-age children. *Language, Speech and Hearing Services in the Schools, 15,* 175–181.

Thrasher, S., & Anderson, G. (1988). The West Indian family: Treatment challenges. *Social Casework: Journal of Contemporary Social Work, March,* 171–176.

Thurnstone, L. L. (1938). *Primary mental abilities.* Psychometrika Monographs, 1.

Thurstone, L. L. (1924). *The nature of intelligence.* New York: Harcourt Brace.

Triandis, H. (1987). Some major dimensions of cultural variation in client populations. In P. Pedersen (Ed.), *Handbook of cross-cultural counseling and therapy* (pp. 21–28). New York: Praeger.

Triandis, H., & Brislin, R. (1984). Cross cultural psychology. *American Psychologist, September,* 1006–1009.

Trinidad plans to fight deportation. (1991, September 16). *Regional Newspaper for the North Eastern Caribbean*, p. 2.

Troike, R. (1968). Social dialects and language learning: Implications for TESOL. *TESOL Quarterly, 2(3)*, 176–180.

Tseng, W., Xu, D., Ebata, K., Hsu, J., & Cul, Y. (1986). Diagnostic pattern for neuroses among China, Japan and America. *American Journal of Psychiatry, 143,* 1010–1014.

Tucker, J. A. (1980). *Nineteen steps for assuring non-biased placement of students in special education.* Reston, VA: ERIC Clearinghouse on Handicapped and Gifted Children.

U.S. Department of Commerce News. (1989, October 12). (Census Bureau Press Release). Hispanic Population surpasses 20 million mark; grows by 39 percent, census bureau reports. (CB 89-58).

U.S. Department of Education. (1992). *The condition of bilingual education in the nation: A report to the Congress and the President.* Washington, DC: Author.

U.S. Department of Education. (1995). *Individuals with Disabilities Education Act Amendments of 1995.*

Valencia, R., Henderson, R., & Rankin, R. (1981). Relationship of family constellation and schooling to intellectual performance of Mexican American children. *Journal of Educational Psychology, 73(4),* 524–532.

Valere-Meredith, J. (1983). *Factors involved in the pidginization process of the English negative system.* Unpublished manuscript.

Valere-Meredith. J. (1985). *Problems in the methodology in the teaching of English as a second dialect.* Unpublished manuscript.

Valere-Meredith. J. (1989). *Teaching English as a second dialect for illiterate West Indians in Canada.* Unpublished manuscript.

Vandenberg, S. G. (1965). Multivariate analysis of twin differences. In S. G. Vandenberg, *Methods and goals in human behavior genetics.* New York: Academic Press.

Vasquez-Nuttal, E., Goldman, P., & Landurand, P. (1983). *A study of mainstreamed limited English proficient handicapped students in bilingual education.* Newton, MA: Vasquez-Nuttall Associates.

Vaughn, B. E., Block, J. E., & Block, J. (1988). Parental agreement on child-rearing during early childhood and the psychological characteristics of adolescents. *Child Development, 59,* 1020–1033.

Velasquez, R., Gonzales, M., Butcher, J., Castillo-Canez, I., Apodaca, J. X., & Chavira, D. (1997). Use of the MMPI-2 with Chicanos: Strategies for counselors. *Journal of Multicultural Counseling and Development, 25,* 107–120.

Vernon, P. E. (1982). *The abilities and achievements of Orientals in North America.* Academic Press.

Vygotsky, L. S. (1978). *Mind in society: The development of higher psychological processes.* Cambridge, MA: Harvard University Press.

Walberg, H. J., Bakalis, M. J. Bast, J. L., & Baer, S. (1988). *We can rescue our children.* Chicago: Heartland Institute.

Walker, J. (1984). *The West Indians in Canada.* Ottawa, Canada: Keystone Printing and Lithographing Ltd.

Wallace, G., Larsen, S.C., & Elksnin, L. K. (1982). *Educational assessment of learning problems: Testing for teaching* (2nd Ed.). Boston: Allyn and Bacon.

Walter, R. (1983). *The groundings with my brothers.* London: Bogle-L'Ouverture Publications Ltd.

Waters, A. M. (1984). *Race, class, and political symbols.* New Brunswick, NJ: Transaction Books.

Watson, D. L., Northcutt, L., & Rydell, L. (February 1989). Teaching bilingual students successfully. *Educational Leadership, 42,* 59–61.

Wechsler, D. (1958). *The measurement and appraisal of adult intelligence* (4th ed.). Baltimore, MD: Williams & Wilkins.

Weidman, H. (1979). Falling-out: A diagnostic and treatment problem viewed from a transcultural perspective. *Social Science and Medicine, 13B,* 95–112.

Welsing, F. C. (1974). The Cress theory of color confrontation. *The Black Scholar, May.*

Werner, O., & Campbell, D. T. (1970). Translating, working through interpreters and the problem of decentering. In R. Naroll & R. Cohen (Eds.), *A handbook of method in cultural anthropology* (pp. 398–420). New York: The Natural History Press.

Westbrook, B., & Sanford, E. (1991). The validity of career maturity attitude measures among Black and white high school students. Special issue: Career development of racial and ethnic minorities. *Career Development Quarterly, 39(3),* 199–208.

Whimbey, A. (1975). *Intelligence can be taught.* New York: Dutton Press.

Whitaker, C. (1986). The West Indian influence. *Ebony, 41(7),* 135–144.

White, S. & Tharp, R. G. (1988, April). Questioning a wait-time: A cross-cultural analysis. *Paper presented at the annual meeting of the American Educational Research Association,* New Orleans.

Whitehurst, G., Fischel, J., Lonigan, C., Valdez-Menchaca, M., Arnold, D., & Smith, M. (1991). Treatment of early expressive language delay: If, when, and how. *Topics in Language Disorders, 11(4),* 55–68.

Whiting, B. (1976). The problem of the packaged variable. In K. Riegel & J. Meacham (Eds.), *The developing individual in a changing world* (pp. 303–309). Chicago, Aldine.

Wiggins, G. (1989). A true test: Toward more authentic and equitable assessment. *Phi Delta Kappan, 70,* 703–713.

Wilen, D. K., & Sweeting, V. M. C. (1986). Assessment of limited English proficient Hispanic students. *School Psychology Review, 15(1),* 59–75.

Williams, E. (1967). *Capitalism and slavery.* London: Lowe & Brydone Printers Ltd.

Williams, E. (1981). *Forge from the love of liberty.* Trinidad and Jamaica: Longman Caribbean.

Williams, R. (1970). Danger: Testing and dehumanizing black children. *Clinical Child Psychology Newsletter, 9(1),* 5–6.

Williams, R. (1971). Abuses and misuses in testing black children. *Washington University Magazine, 41(3),* 34–37.

Williams, R. (1975). The BITCH-100: A culture-specific test. *Journal of Afro-American Issues, 3,* 103–106.

Williams, R. (1980). Scientific racism and IQ: The silent mugging of the black community. *Psychology Today, 7(12),* 32–41.

Wittkower, E. D. (1964). Spirit possession in Haitian voodoo ceremonies. *Acta Psychother, 12,* 72–80.

Wober, M. (1974). Towards an understanding of the Kiganda concept of intelligence. In J. W. Berry & P. R. Dasen (Eds.), *Culture and cognition: Readings in cross-cultural psychology.* Methuen.

Wrenn, C. G. (1985). Afterward: The culturally encapsulated counselor revisited. In P. Pedersen (Ed.), *Handbook of cross-cultural counseling and therapy* (pp. 323–329). Westport, CT: Greenwood Press.

Yee, A. H. (1983). *Ethnicity and race: Psychology Perspectives.*

Yekwai, D. (1988). *British racism: Miseducation and the Afrikan child.* London: Karnak House.

Young, L., & Bagley, C. (1979). *Identity, self-esteem and evaluation of color and ethnicity in young children in Jamaica and London.* Paper presented at the 3rd annual conference of the Society of Caribbean Studies, London.

Zuckerman, M. (1990). Some dubious premises in research and theory on racial differences: Scientific, social, and ethical issues. *American Psychologist, 45,* 1297–1303.

BIOSKETCH OF AUTHORS

Sharon-ann Gopaul-McNicol, Ph.D.
Dr. Sharon-ann Gopaul-McNicol, originally from Trinidad and Tobago, West Indies, is an international expert in multicultural assessment. She is the assistant director of accreditation at the American Psychological Association. She is the former director of the school psychology program at Howard University and a licensed clinical and school psychologist. Over the past ten years, Dr. Gopaul-McNicol, has assessed children both nationally and internationally, including London, several countries from the English-, Spanish- and French-speaking Caribbean. The author of eight cross-cultural books and several journal articles, Dr. Gopaul-McNicol has given presentations throughout the world both on electronic media and at various international conferences.

Dr. Eleanor Armour-Thomas, Ed.D.
Dr. Eleanor Armour-Thomas, originally from Trinidad and Tobago, West Indies, is professor of educational psychology in the department of secondary education at Queens College and the Ph.D. Program in Educational Psychology at the Graduate School and University Center of the City University of New York. Her co-authored books and scholarly publications center around assessment of cognitive competencies underlying student and teacher performance and the role of culture on human behavior. She is currently the chair of the department of secondary education and has conducted policy studies on teaching for the National Commission on Teaching and Americas Future and the College Entrance Examination Board.

Both authors have developed the bio-cultural model to assessing intelligence, the model that has served to guide the development of this book, and that is used both nationally and internationally.

INDEX